100 Questions & Answers About Infertility

Second Edition

John David Gordon, MD
Clinical Professor
The George Washington University
Department of Obstetrics and Gynecology
Co-Director
Dominion Fertility
Arlington, VA

Michael DiMattina, MD
Clinical Associate Professor
Georgetown University School of Medicine
Department of Obstetrics and Gynecology
Director
Dominion Fertility
Arlington, VA

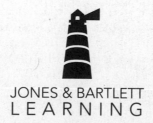

JONES & BARTLETT
LEARNING

World Headquarters
Jones & Bartlett Learning
40 Tall Pine Drive
Sudbury, MA 01776
978-443-5000
info@jblearning.com
www.jblearning.com

Jones & Bartlett Learning
Canada
6339 Ormindale Way
Mississauga, Ontario L5V 1J2
Canada

Jones & Bartlett Learning
International
Barb House, Barb Mews
London W6 7PA
United Kingdom

Jones & Bartlett Learning books and products are available through most bookstores and online booksellers. To contact Jones & Bartlett Learning directly, call 800-832-0034, fax 978-443-8000, or visit our website, www.jblearning.com.

Substantial discounts on bulk quantities of Jones & Bartlett Learning publications are available to corporations, professional associations, and other qualified organizations. For details and specific discount information, contact the special sales department at Jones & Bartlett Learning via the above contact information or send an email to specialsales@jblearning.com.

The authors, editor, and publisher have made every effort to provide accurate information. However, they are not responsible for errors, omissions, or for any outcomes related to the use of the contents of this book and take no responsibility for the use of the products and procedures described. Treatments and side effects described in this book may not be applicable to all people; likewise, some people may require a dose or experience a side effect that is not described herein. Drugs and medical devices are discussed that may have limited availability controlled by the Food and Drug Administration (FDA) for use only in a research study or clinical trial. Research, clinical practice, and government regulations often change the accepted standard in this field. When consideration is being given to use of any drug in the clinical setting, the healthcare provider or reader is responsible for determining FDA status of the drug, reading the package insert, and reviewing prescribing information for the most up-to-date recommendations on dose, precautions, and contraindications, and determining the appropriate usage for the product. This is especially important in the case of drugs that are new or seldom used.

Production Credits
Executive Publisher: Christopher Davis
Production Director: Amy Rose
Editorial Assistant: Sara Cameron
Senior Production Editor: Daniel Stone
Associate Marketing Manager: Katie Hennessy
Manufacturing and Inventory Control Supervisor:
  Amy Bacus
Composition: Glyph International
Printing and Binding: Malloy, Inc.

Cover Credits
Cover Design: Carolyn Downer
Cover Printing: Malloy, Inc.
Cover Images: Top Left: © Kurhan/
  ShutterStock, Inc.; Top Right: © Monkey
  Business Images/ShutterStock, Inc.;
  Bottom: © Monkey Business Images/
  ShutterStock, Inc.

4491 2078 1/11

Library of Congress Cataloging-in-Publication Data
Gordon, John D. (John David)
  100 questions & answers about infertility/John D. Gordon, Michael
DiMattina.—2nd ed.
    p. cm.
  Includes bibliographical references and index.
  ISBN 978-0-7637-9108-7 (alk. paper)
  1. Infertility—Miscellanea. 2. Infertility—Popular works. I.
DiMattina, Michael. II. Title. III. Title: One hundred questions and answers
about infertility.
  RC899.G67 2011
  616.6'92—dc22

                            2010026643

6048

Printed in the United States of America
14 13 12 11 10   10 9 8 7 6 5 4 3 2 1

Contents

Contents

v

Patients ask me frequently for book recommendations. They want a book that will answer all of their basic questions about infertility. I am only comfortable recommending ones that are up-to-date, comprehensive, and truly honest about the success rates of the various treatments. Most importantly, I need my patients to have as a resource a book to guide them through their journey and to help make the decisions they need to make. They want and need the facts, presented in an understandable and logical fashion.

I read this book cover to cover (and in such detail that I have to admit I actually asked the authors to tweak it here and there to cover things like mind/body and stress to my satisfaction!) because I feel incredibly strongly that those who are experiencing infertility deserve to be well educated. The reproductive system is so complicated that one of the infertility physicians I work with often remarks that it is a miracle any of us were conceived naturally! You don't need to have an advanced degree and you don't have to understand every hormone and gland, but if you are undergoing an infertility workup or treatment, you need to know enough to feel comfortable with the plan your physician is recommending for you.

Most, if not all, of my patients get the vast majority of their information from the Internet, which is fine if that information is accurate. Unfortunately, that is often not the case. Research has shown that more than 50 percent of the medical information found online is not correct. Occasionally I lurk on some of the more popular chat rooms, and I have been disturbed to see some of the myths and exaggerations repeated over and over. It would be so nice if indeed a certain herb could treat high follicle-stimulating hormone (FSH) levels and lead to viable pregnancies. It would be terrific if clomiphene would always work if you just give it enough time or increase the dose enough, but the truth is that a lot of what we find on the Internet is either what people want to believe, or simply someone trying to make money off of your vulnerability.

Fortunately, if you receive treatment from a physician appropriately trained in infertility treatment, you have an excellent chance of becoming a parent. Unfortunately, that physician often doesn't have the time to answer every single one of your questions.

The goal of this text is to give you the background information you need. If you know the basics about infertility, you can use the time you have with your physician to tailor *your* questions to *you*: What is your diagnosis? What is your treatment plan? How does your physician plan to maximize the chances that you will successfully conceive?

Use this book as a weapon against your infertility. I wish you the very best of luck.

Alice D. Domar, PhD
Executive Director
Domar Center for Mind/Body Health
Boston IVF
Assistant Professor of Obstetrics, Gynecology, and
Reproductive Biology, Harvard Medical School
Boston, MA
Author, *Conquering Infertility*

As physicians specializing in reproductive endocrinology and infertility, it has been our privilege to care for thousands of patients over our 35 combined years of clinical practice. In 1978, the birth of the world's first IVF baby, Louise Brown, ushered in a new era in reproductive medicine. What few patients and doctors seem to remember is that Drs. Steptoe and Edwards accomplished this remarkable success by performing IVF in an unstimulated reproductive cycle. The past few years have brought exciting new changes to the practice of infertility. In particular, IVF has begun to swing full circle as we have increasingly incorporated unstimulated, or Natural Cycle IVF, into our practice with gratifying results. Although most US fertility practices do not offer this option, Natural Cycle IVF has been embraced by fertility physicians outside of the United States for many years. Clearly, unstimulated IVF will not replace stimulated cycle IVF, but 30 years after the birth of Louise Brown, it seems an appropriate tribute to that remarkable accomplishment.

Infertility is an emotionally traumatic life event. Although medical progress in the treatment of infertility has been nothing less than astounding, the toll that infertility can take on a couple's or a woman's emotional, spiritual, psychological, and physical well-being can be extreme. Our patients are always our best teachers. We hope that by sharing with you, the reader of this book, some of the frequent questions that we are asked along with our responses, we can help you navigate the voyage ahead as you pursue the evaluation and treatment of infertility.

John David Gordon, MD
Michael DiMattina, MD

First of all, we wish to acknowledge the staff at Dominion Fertility and thank them for all of the outstanding work that they do on behalf of our patients. It is easy to look good when you are supported by such caring individuals. Secondly, we wish to extend our heartfelt thanks to Dr. David Adamson and Dr. Alice Domar for their insightful comments about this manuscript and their kind words in the introduction and the foreword, respectively. In addition, we wish to thank Kristin, Rebecca, and Carol for their participation in this project and for giving a patient's perspective of fertility treatment. Finally, we would like to thank the staff at Jones & Bartlett Learning (especially Sara Cameron, Kathy Richardson, and Chris Davis) for their support and editorial assistance with this project.

John David Gordon, MD
Michael DiMattina, MD

It is a great pleasure to write an introduction to Dr. John David Gordon and Dr. Michael DiMattina's book *100 Questions and Answers About Infertility, Second Edition*. I have known these fine physicians for a long time and know of their commitment to the education of patients who are suffering from infertility.

The obvious barriers for most patients facing infertility are physical problems of the ovaries, uterus, and fallopian tubes; other hormonal problems; sperm problems; and/or multiple other, more complex factors. It is essential for physicians to identify the problems causing infertility so that effective, individualized treatments can be recommended to each patient. However, patients cannot give themselves their best chance to conceive a baby unless they understand the proposed treatments and can communicate clearly with their physician.

Every treatment has differences in financial cost, time duration, medical risk, and emotional stress. These factors can be perceived very differently by patients depending on their age, duration of infertility, prior treatments, insurance coverage, causes of infertility, religious or moral values, and emotional commitment to fertility treatment. It is impossible for patients to make appropriate choices unless they have a good understanding of their treatment choices. Knowledge is power, especially for infertility patients.

However, it is very difficult to get good information today. Indeed, while many wonderful advantages have been brought about by the Internet and other sources, we are overwhelmed with inaccurate, incorrect, or even purposely misleading information, often written by self-described "medical experts" or those with a limited personal experience of infertility. The information gained from such sources often provides interesting reading, but is usually of little value—and is potentially harmful—to patients trying to make decisions about their infertility treatment. Harm can come from wasting time, money, or emotional resources on treatments that are not the best choice, may not even be effective, and may be risky.

That is where a book like this one becomes so valuable. Dr. Gordon and Dr. DiMattina have written a book that answers 100 commonly asked questions in a straightforward and easily understandable manner. They have identified these questions based on years of experience with patients. They have developed their answers based on their experience and success, and with an understanding of scientific studies in the literature, evidence-based medicine, and national practice guidelines developed by the American Society for Reproductive Medicine. Furthermore, they have been careful to provide a balanced perspective of the advantages and disadvantages of different treatments. This helps patients understand that often more than one approach may be possible and that their own financial and emotional situations are important considerations in deciding the best treatment for them.

I believe that all infertility patients will benefit from reading this very well-written and comprehensive book. This book answers the questions infertility patients need to know, and this knowledge will help them increase their chances of having a baby. With my sincere wishes for good reading and good luck!

David Adamson, MD, FRCSC, FACOG, FACS
Director, Fertility Physicians of Northern California
Adjunct Clinical Professor, Stanford University
Associate Clinical Professor, University of California
at San Francisco

PART ONE

The Basics

How does normal human reproduction work?

What is infertility?

How common is infertility?

More...

1. How does normal human reproduction work?

Normal human female reproduction depends on the correct functioning of four components of a woman's body: the brain, the **ovary**, the **fallopian tube**, and the **uterus**. At the time of her birth, a woman's ovary contains all of the eggs that she will ever have. These eggs are contained within fluid-filled sacs called **follicles**.

Every month, the brain sends out a signal from the **pituitary gland** (a gland located at the base of the brain) stimulating the follicles to grow. Not surprisingly, this hormone is called **follicle-stimulating hormone (FSH)**. Under the influence of FSH, a group of follicles begins to grow, but by the fifth day of the reproductive cycle a single dominant follicle has already been selected. This dominant follicle may be either on the right ovary or the left ovary.

As it grows, the follicle produces an important steroid hormone called **estrogen**. Estrogen causes the lining of the uterus (**endometrium**) to thicken in anticipation of the eventual **implantation** of an embryo.

By mid-cycle, this follicle has grown to a diameter of 20 to 22 mm. At this time, the brain releases a second hormone, called **luteinizing hormone (LH)**, from the pituitary gland. LH is the trigger that induces **ovulation**.

Approximately 36 hours after the LH surge, the follicle releases the egg. It is the job of the fallopian tube to trap the egg. If the fallopian tube fails to catch the egg, then pregnancy cannot occur.

During intercourse, tens of millions of sperm are deposited in the woman's vagina when her male partner reaches

Ovary

A female reproductive organ that contains eggs and produces reproductive hormones.

Fallopian tube

The conduit that serves as an incubator following release and fertilization of the egg.

Uterus

The pear-shaped organ that contains a growing pregnancy.

Follicles

Fluid-filled structures within the ovary that contain an egg.

Pituitary gland

An organ located at the base of the brain that controls several of the other hormone-producing glands.

Follicle-stimulating hormone (FSH)

A protein hormone that promotes the growth and development of follicles, leading eventually to ovulation.

orgasm and ejaculates. While the egg is safely held within the fallopian tube, these sperm swim from the vagina, into the cervix, through the uterus, and up into the fallopian tube, where **fertilization** occurs. (see **Figure 1**). Normally, the growing embryo travels through the fallopian tube for 5 days after fertilization, at which point it reaches the uterus. (An embryo that remains trapped within the fallopian tube is called a tubal pregnancy or **ectopic pregnancy**, and can be a life-threatening condition.) The embryo divides many times along the way, and by the time it reaches the uterus, it has grown to hundreds of cells and is called a **blastocyst**.

Once the egg is released from the ovary, the follicle (now called a **corpus luteum**) continues to produce estrogen

Estrogen

A steroid hormone produced within the growing follicle that induces growth of the endometrium.

Endometrium

The tissue that lines the uterine cavity and is shed each month with a woman's period.

Implantation

The attachment of the early embryo to the endometrial lining of the uterus.

The Basics

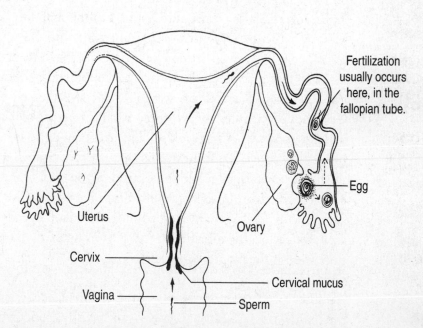

Fertilization usually occurs here, in the fallopian tube.

Egg

Uterus

Ovary

Cervix

Cervical mucus

Vagina

Sperm

Figure 1   Female reproductive organs. Solid arrows indicate the path sperm must travel to reach the egg. Dotted arrows indicate the path of the egg. The fertilized egg continues traveling through the fallopian tube to the uterus.

Source: © 2006 American Society for Reproductive Medicine.

Luteinizing hormone (LH)

A pituitary hormone that induces ovulation in a mature follicle.

Ovulation

The release of an egg from an ovarian follicle.

Fertilization

The process by which an egg and a sperm combine and create an embryo.

Ectopic pregnancy

A pregnancy located outside the uterine cavity, usually in the fallopian tube.

Blastocyst

A stage in embryo development reached 5 days after fertilization.

Corpus luteum

The hormone-producing ovarian cyst that forms from the follicle after it releases the egg.

Progesterone

A steroid hormone produced by the ovary necessary for successful embryo implantation.

Infertility

The inability of a couple to conceive after 12 months of unprotected intercourse.

and begins to produce a new hormone: **progesterone**. Progesterone induces changes in the estrogen-primed endometrium, allowing implantation of the embryo and thus permitting pregnancy to occur. In the absence of a pregnancy, the levels of estrogen and progesterone both fall 2 weeks after ovulation and a menstrual period ensues, shedding the lining of the uterus. Menstrual flow lasts approximately 3 to 5 days in most women.

Overall, human beings are not very fertile, with maximum pregnancy rates of only 20% to 25% per cycle during the years of peak fertility (the second and third decades of life).

2. What is infertility?

Approximately 80% to 85% of couples who are trying to become pregnant will successfully conceive within a year. Thus, **infertility** is commonly defined as the inability to achieve a pregnancy within 12 months of unprotected intercourse. However, certain patients may have recognized factors that preclude normal conception. For them, the 12-month period of waiting makes little sense. Common examples of women with such problems include those who have extremely irregular periods, a history of severe **endometriosis**, a history of previous tubal pregnancies, or other anatomical factors that would clearly lead to diminished fertility. Since fertility declines significantly as a woman ages, couples are encouraged to seek evaluation for infertility after 6 months of no contraception if the woman is older than age 35.

Another problem related to reproduction is recurrent pregnancy loss. Many women can readily conceive, only to suffer repeated pregnancy losses (see Questions 92–99). These women represent a special subset of those who are unable to successfully reproduce and should be evaluated by a medical professional.

3. How common is infertility?

Infertility is an extraordinarily common disorder. An estimated 25% of all women will experience an episode of infertility during their lifetime. In the United States, infertility currently affects about 6.1 million women and their partners. The percentage of reproductive-age women who report problems in successfully conceiving and maintaining a pregnancy varies with age. In the youngest segment of the population, approximately 10% to 15% are affected by this problem. Among women older than age 35, however, more than one-third report diminished fertility. The rates of pregnancy loss are also related to a woman's age, with the rate of miscarriage exceeding 50% in women older than age 40.

Endometriosis

The presence of endometrial tissue outside of the endometrial cavity.

The Basics

Kristin comments:

When you're in the throes of infertility, desperately wanting a child while seemingly everybody around you gets pregnant on their "first try," you wonder if you're the only one who can't get pregnant. My husband and I have been very open about our fertility problems, and once I really started to share our story with friends and acquaintances I discovered I was not alone . . . far from it. I have created amazing friendships with other "infertiles" I have met through Internet communities, reading blogs, and even support groups in my area.

4. Is infertility becoming more common?

A common misperception is that infertility is becoming more common. In fact, the infertility rate has held relatively stable over the years. Instead, two major factors account for the increased utilization of fertility services.

The first of these factors is simply the greater availability of the services themselves. Prior to the 1978 birth of Louise Brown, the world's first baby conceived through

In vitro fertilization (IVF)

A fertility treatment in which an egg is placed with a sperm cell in a laboratory culture dish, cultured for several days, and subsequently placed into the uterus.

Ovulation induction

The use of fertility medications to restore normal ovulation in a woman who does not have regular cycles.

More than 100,000 cycles of ART are performed in the United States every year.

in vitro fertilization (IVF), the options available to treat an infertile couple were limited to tubal microsurgery and ovulation induction with medications such as clomiphene citrate (Clomid). With the development of advanced reproductive technologies (ART), the techniques used to treat infertile couples have become both much more successful and more accessible. Fertility providers now practice throughout nearly all urban centers in the continental United States, with more than 400 IVF clinics reporting their success rates through the Society for Assisted Reproductive Technologies (SART) and the Centers for Disease Control and Prevention (CDC). Statistics from all reporting IVF clinics are available at http://www.cdc.gov/ART/index.htm.

The second factor accounting for the increased use of fertility services is the trend toward delayed childbearing. Over the last generation, a significant number of women have deferred childbearing while they pursued advanced academic careers or entered the workplace. Unfortunately, female reproductive capacity drops from a peak in the second and third decades of life so that, by the age of 40 years, there is a marked reduction in fertility and an increased risk of miscarriage.

Finally, the stigma associated with fertility treatments themselves has also eased in recent years, prompting more couples to seek out such help. Previously, couples who were seeking fertility treatments often found themselves beset by a bewildering array of options and knew few other couples with whom they could discuss the range of treatments. Today, more than 100,000 cycles of ART are performed in the United States every year. Given that 1% of all U.S. births are now the result of fertility treatments, most couples probably know someone with a successful outcome from fertility treatments.

The current explosion of information available through the Internet and through organizations such as the American Society for Reproductive Medicine (ASRM), RESOLVE, and the American Fertility Association has allowed patients to better understand fertility-related problems and seek appropriate care. A number of states have implemented mandates that guarantee varying levels of insurance coverage for fertility-related procedures, which has had the effect of easing the financial burden for couples who seek out this type of care.

Kristin comments:

When I started discussing my fertility problems with my mother, she opened up about her own struggles to conceive my brother and me. While she did eventually get pregnant on her own, it took her over 2 years to conceive me and about the same amount of time to conceive my brother. She said that nobody really talked about infertility when she was trying to get pregnant and the fertility options were minimal. My mother was an only child because my grandmother could never become pregnant again despite years of trying. I would guess that both my grandmother and my mother had the same infertility diagnosis as I do—PCOS [polycystic ovarian syndrome]—but in their childbearing years it was not commonly diagnosed and treatments were either nonexistent or limited.

The Basics

PART TWO

The Fertility Evaluation and Treatment Basics

What are typical causes of infertility?

What tests will we have to undergo as part of a fertility evaluation?

How expensive are infertility treatments?

More . . .

5. Who should evaluate the infertile couple? Do I need to see a reproductive endocrinologist?

In many cases, the routine fertility evaluation can be conducted by an obstetrician/gynecologist, or a family practitioner. Certain tests can easily be ordered and interpreted by physicians in the first two specialties, but a **reproductive endocrinologist** (RE) may be required to interpret advanced testing and provide the most accurate counseling. Women who are more than 34 years old may elect to immediately consult with a reproductive endocrinologist.

Although all physicians trained in obstetrics and gynecology are exposed to the specialty of reproductive endocrinology and infertility, this training may by cursory at best. On the other hand, a reproductive endocrinologist (RE) is a physician who specializes in the treatment of reproductive disorders and infertility. A physician specializing in reproductive endocrinology undergoes 4 years of training in general obstetrics and gynecology following his or her completion of medical school. At the end of these 4 years of internship and residency (which includes exposure to normal and high-risk obstetrics, gynecology, gynecologic oncology, and reproductive endocrinology and infertility) a physician may then apply for an additional 3-year fellowship in reproductive endocrinology and infertility. There are usually only 25–35 fellowship positions available each year, so competition can be intense. After completing these 7 years of training, the physician takes a series of written and oral examinations to become board-certified in this specialty. Although not all practitioners of reproductive endocrinology and infertility have undergone formal fellowship-level training, the majority have, and this training includes both clinical and basic science experience.

Reproductive endocrinologist

A physician who specializes in disorders of reproduction, including infertility.

There are several professional organizations for physicians who are interested in the treatment of the infertile couple, including the American Society of Reproductive Medicine (ASRM) and the Society for Reproductive Endocrinology and Infertility (SREI). Any physician who is interested in infertility may join ASRM, but members of SREI must be board eligible or board certified in reproductive endocrinology and infertility. Both of these organizations maintain websites that allow patients to identify local specialists (www.asrm.org; www.socrei.org).

Members of SREI must be board eligible or board certified in reproductive endocrinology and infertility.

Carol comments:

I began discussions with my gynecologist at age 34 regarding my lack of success at getting pregnant. He put me on a plan that seemed to represent a pretty standard process of elimination. First, I did the basal body temperature charting for 3 months to determine if I was ovulating; then, I spent 3 months on Clomid with no success. Looking back on it now, I question his resistance to send me directly to an RE for further evaluation given my age and what the ovulation charting had revealed. Don't be afraid to push your doctors. I wish I would have pushed harder to get things moving.

6. How do I choose a fertility clinic?

Choosing a fertility doctor for your care may be the single most important factor that leads to a successful pregnancy, so choose carefully.

Many patients are referred to us by their OB/GYN, friends, relatives, former patients, news articles, or through the Internet. But the one common denominator we have routinely observed with the sophisticated patient is that she is well prepared before coming for her initial office visit or she quickly becomes informed and knowledgeable before we begin any treatments. Patients often say to us, "I checked you out before making this appointment." Of course, we are always flattered by such comments, and we anticipate that this patient will ask all of the important questions and make an intelligent decision regarding her treatment options. She will also probably experience less stress during the evaluation and treatment process, as she has developed a better knowledge base and understanding of what to expect.

All fertility clinics come with a unique flavor of their own. Some are run by a solo practitioner, others by two- to six-member groups, while others are clinics with more than 15 doctors. Regardless of the size of the group, be sure you are getting the attention and treatments you desire and deserve. You should never feel like a number with a revolving door of doctors.

A caring doctor will always welcome any and all questions and will take the time to answer them in a way that you can understand.

Of course, patients are not doctors and will not have the knowledge or experience of a reproductive endocrinologist, but a caring doctor will always welcome any and all questions and will take the time to answer them in a way that you can understand. We view patients as our partners, and once we understand what they are willing or not willing to do, we can devise a treatment plan that offers hope without subjecting them to any unnecessary additional stress.

Other Things to Consider

Statistics, statistics, statistics: You want a baby, so choose a fertility clinic with good success rates. However, a wise man once said: "There are lies, damn lies, and statistics." So, how does one determine what to make of these statistics? In truth, there is no easy answer.

Clinics that are more selective can inflate their success rates, while those that have a different philosophy may suffer the consequences even though they have an excellent program. For example, clinics that encourage elective single **embryo transfer** (eSET) or that offer unstimulated or **Natural Cycle IVF** may demonstrate lower clinical pregnancy rates because fewer embryos are transferred. Yet, in fact, such clinics that routinely transfer one or two embryos may have the best IVF programs. When considering a clinic, it is important to know what your specific chances for success will be within that clinic.

If there is one yardstick with which to compare clinics, then we recommend examining the pregnancy rate using donor eggs. In this patient population, the pregnancy rates should be very high. A low donor egg pregnancy rate may be concerning. All clinics should have a good pool of young egg donors and a recipient population that is fairly similar, allowing for better comparison of clinics.

Advertising may be misleading. Obviously, a practice with 10 to 20 doctors will produce more total babies than a medical practice with only 2 to 6 fertility doctors, but the pregnancy rates may be equivalent (as can be seen in Figure 41 of Appendix B). Individuals should evaluate the clinic statistics and obtain a good understanding and feel for what their specific chances for pregnancy will be per treatment. Patients may also evaluate the clinic's success by reviewing IVF statistics at the Centers for Disease Control and Prevention (www.cdc.gov/ART/index.htm/).

Experience: Experience of the clinic, in our opinion, may be one of the most important factors when deciding

Embryo transfer

The placement of embryos created via in vitro fertilization into the uterus or, more rarely, the fallopian tube.

Natural Cycle IVF

A type of IVF treatment that does not use any fertility medications but rather uses the single egg that is normally produced in a typical reproductive cycle.

The Fertility Evaluation and Treatment Basics

which doctor and which clinic to consult for fertility care. One should ask how long the doctors have been performing various treatment procedures. It is also important to know whether or not cutting edge procedures are either being offered or are being developed in the practice.

Subspecialty board certification: Most doctors practicing in the field of in vitro fertilization and infertility are subspecialty board certified in reproductive endocrinology and infertility. Evidence of this certification can be found by going to the Society for Reproductive Endocrinology's website, which lists doctors who are subspecialty certified in reproductive endocrinology and infertility. Additionally, patients may find it beneficial to check if their doctor has a faculty position at one of the local medical universities or actively participates in the teaching of medical students and residents in their locality.

Availability and accessibility of doctors: It is important that you have access to your doctor in order to have your questions answered and needs addressed. Evaluate whether or not the availability and accessibility of the doctor is an easy process or a difficult one when making decisions as to where to seek care. The friendliness and helpfulness of the staff will also give you a feel for the character of the practice.

Cost: It is always important to get the total cost. Factor in extra expenses such as the fertility drugs, which can cost thousands of dollars; **intracytoplasmic sperm injection (ICSI)**; assisted embryo hatching; embryo **cryopreservation**; and **preimplantation genetic diagnosis (PGD)**. These drugs and procedures can quickly increase the overall cost for treatment.

It is important that you have access to your doctor.

Intracytoplasmic sperm injection (ICSI)

The injection of a sperm into an egg, in IVF cases when fertilization might not otherwise occur.

Cryopreservation

Freezing of sperm, eggs, or embryos so as to preserve them for use at a later date.

Preimplantation genetic diagnosis (PGD)

Evaluation of the genetic status of an embryo prior to its implantation, usually through the removal of 1 to 2 cells at the 8-cell stage of development. The isolated cells can then be analyzed for specific chromosomal conditions and other genetic disorders.

A word of caution: In general, Internet chat rooms and bulletin/message boards may be dangerous places for seeking advice regarding finding an infertility doctor. Be careful what you hear online, as it always represents just one half of the story. It is far better for you to do your own homework and research than to rely on information provided by others, which may be based on misleading impressions or experiences. Patients reporting on their experience with a given clinic or doctor may represent both extremes of the spectrum.

7. What are typical causes of infertility?

The causes of infertility are wide ranging but can be examined in light of the reproductive cycle described in Question 1. (See **Table 1**.) In general, the causes of infertility can be equally divided between the male and female partners in a couple.

The causes of infertility can be equally divided between the male and female partners in a couple.

Table 1   **Diagnoses Among Couples Who Had ART Cycles Using Fresh Nondonor Eggs or Embryos,* 2006**

Cause of Infertility	%
Endometriosis	5.1
Ovulatory dysfunction	6.4
Other causes	8.3
Diminished ovarian reserve	9.2
Tubal factor	9.8
Multiple factors, female only	11.3
Uterine factor	1.4
Multiple factors (female + male)	18.3
Male factor	18.3
Unexplained cause	12.0

*Total does not equal 100% due to rounding.

Source: Adapted from the Centers for Disease Control and Prevention. 2006 Assisted Reproductive Technology Success Rates, December 2009.

Half of all infertility cases, therefore, involve problems with the sperm of the male partner. Unfortunately, functional tests for sperm competence (the ability of sperm to fertilize an egg) are not available leaving us to rely upon the descriptive components of the **semen analysis**. A complete semen analysis should include the total number of sperm (concentration), the percentage of those sperm that are moving (motility), and the shape of those sperm (morphology).

Many factors can reduce the female partner's ability to conceive. For example, a woman may have anatomical problems related to the fallopian tubes, uterus, and peritoneal structures within the pelvis such as **adhesions** or endometriosis. Problems with ovulation are very common in infertile patients, and women with irregular periods may suffer from a common disorder such as **polycystic ovarian syndrome (PCOS)**. Another major fertility factor is reproductive aging. Peak fertility occurs when a woman is in her twenties, and it declines significantly during her thirties and forties. The rate of decline increases after the age of 35 as is evident in decreased IVF pregnancy rates and decreased embryo implantation rates in this age group.

8. What tests will we have to undergo as part of a fertility evaluation?

The basic infertility evaluation consists of a handful of tests. The woman typically undergoes a **transvaginal ultrasound**, hormone blood tests, and an assessment of the fallopian tubes and uterus (by x-ray or by laparoscopic surgery). The man gets off relatively easily as he usually only undergoes a semen analysis.

Transvaginal ultrasound allows the physician to assess the appearance of the uterus and the ovaries. During

---

Semen analysis

A laboratory test used to assess male fertility. It usually includes evaluation of the sperm volume, pH, concentration, motility and morphology in a sample.

Adhesions

Bands of fibrous tissue that can bind reproductive organs, thereby reducing a woman's fertility.

Polycystic ovarian syndrome (PCOS)

A common gynecologic disorder often leading to irregular periods and infertility.

Transvaginal ultrasound

An imaging technique that uses sound waves produced by a wand-like probe placed within the vagina.

this examination, the physician may discover uterine abnormalities such as **fibroids** (benign growths of the muscle of the uterus) or uterine polyps (benign growths of the lining of the uterus). **Ultrasonography** can also identify the location of the ovaries and determine the number of follicles present (**antral follicle count**), which correlates with the woman's response to fertility medications. In addition, examination of the ovaries may reveal the presence of abnormal ovarian cysts such as **endometriomas**, dermoid cysts, or—in rare cases—precancerous and cancerous lesions.

In addition to the routine vaginal ultrasound, an assessment of the fallopian tubes and the uterine cavity is appropriate when the woman is having trouble conceiving. This examination is usually accomplished through a **hysterosalpingogram** (HSG: see **Figure 2**), an x-ray test that is performed under fluoroscopy by a

Fibroids

Benign growths of the connective tissue of the uterus.

Ultrasonography

A noninvasive imaging technology that uses sound waves to create images of various structures in the body.

Antral follicle count

The number of resting follicles seen on ultrasound early in a woman's cycle.

Endometriomas

An ovarian cyst that is filled with chocolate-colored fluid as a result of endometriosis growing within the ovary.

The Fertility Evaluation and Treatment Basics

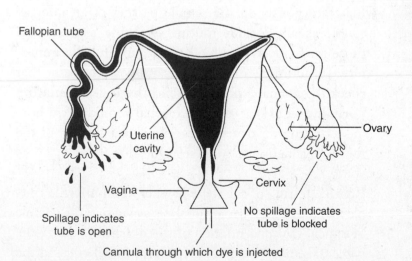

Fallopian tube
Uterine cavity
Ovary
Vagina
Cervix
Spillage indicates tube is open
No spillage indicates tube is blocked
Cannula through which dye is injected

Figure 2   HSG, a procedure to determine if the fallopian tubes are open or blocked.

Source: © 2006 American Society for Reproductive Medicine.

17

**Hysterosalpingo-
gram**

An x-ray procedure to
assess the fallopian
tubes for patency.

Laparoscopy

An outpatient surgi-
cal procedure that
uses a telescope and
video monitor to
visualize the internal
organs.

Hysteroscopy

A procedure allowing
visualization of the
uterine cavity with a
small fiber-optic
telescope.

Prolactin

A hormone produced
by the anterior pitu-
itary that stimulates
breast milk
production.

**Thyroid-
stimulating
hormone (TSH)**

A hormone produced
by the pituitary gland
that stimulates the
production of thyroid
hormone from the
thyroid gland.

Ovarian reserve

The fertility potential
of a woman as deter-
mined by both the
number of her ovar-
ian follicles and the
health of the eggs
located within those
follicles.

gynecologist, a reproductive endocrinologist or a radiologist. Although it may sometimes cause mild uterine
cramping, the vast majority of patients tolerate this
procedure without difficulty. The individual physician
performing this test can make a huge difference in the
experience for a typical patient. For example, we utilize
a soft catheter which is held in place against the cervix
but is not actually passed into the uterine cavity. The use
of this instrument, rather than a balloon type catheter
that must be introduced through the cervix and into
the uterus, can markedly reduce patient discomfort
with this test. Similarly, only a small volume of dye is
needed to fill the uterus and fallopian tubes. Excessive
pressure and volume of dye can lead to much greater
cramping and rarely improves the diagnostic accuracy
of the test.

Alternatives to the hysterosalpingogram include **laparoscopy** and **hysteroscopy**; these outpatient surgical
procedures are described in Questions 11 and 12.

Laboratory tests on the female partner of an infertile
couple usually include routine screening tests such as
those for blood type, blood count, and rubella immu-
nity. In addition, most physicians perform tests that
check the woman's **prolactin** and **thyroid-stimulating
hormone (TSH)** levels. Additional reproductive hormone testing for **ovarian reserve** is usually part of the
routine evaluation as well (see Question 9).

Routine testing of the male partner of an infertile couple includes a basic semen analysis evaluating the volume
of semen, the concentration of sperm (sperm count), the
percentage of moving sperm (**sperm motility**), and the
percentage of normally shaped sperm (**sperm morphology**). (See **Table 2**.) Although some clinics perform

Table 2   Components of the Routine Semen Analysis

Parameter	Reference Value
Volume	1.5–5.0 mL (pH, 7.2)
Concentration	> 20 million/mL
Total motile count	10 million
Motility	> 50%
Normal morphology	> 30% normal (World Health Organization, 1999) > 14% normal (Kruger and Coetzee, 1999)
Indirect immuno-bead assay (sperm antibodies)	≥ 20%

Source: Adapted from World Health Organization. *WHO Laboratory Manual for the Examination of Human Semen and Semen–Cervical Mucus Interaction*. New York: Cambridge University Press, 1999.

additional sperm function tests, such as the **acrosome reaction** and **hypo-osmotic swelling test**, the overall benefit of these two tests remains somewhat controversial. Both of these tests attempt to predict the functional ability of the sperm in terms of its ability to fertilize an egg. Ultimately, however, the best evidence of normal sperm function is a recent pregnancy or normal fertilization during a cycle of IVF.

Tests to detect the presence of **antisperm antibodies** in the blood of the female partner or coating the individual sperm may sometimes be recommended. Female antisperm antibodies may cause infertility that is best treated by IVF. Antisperm antibodies present on the sperm themselves may inhibit normal fertilization. In such cases, collecting a semen sample in media for use in

---

The Fertility Evaluation and Treatment Basics

Sperm motility

The movement of sperm when viewed under a microscope.

Sperm morphology

The shape and outward appearance of the sperm when viewed under a microscope.

Acrosome reaction

A test to assess the biochemical changes on the head of the sperm that may predict the ability of the sperm to fertilize an egg.

Hypo-osmotic swelling test

A sperm test that evaluates the integrity of the outer membrane of the sperm as a means to predict the sperm's fertilizing ability.

The best evidence of normal sperm function is a recent pregnancy or normal fertilization during a cycle of IVF.

Antisperm antibodies

Proteins that can lead to infertility by impairing fertilization or enhancing sperm destruction within the female reproductive tract.

Artificial insemination

A group of fertility procedures involving the introduction of sperm into the female reproductive tract without intercourse.

Diminished ovarian reserve

The inability to respond appropriately to fertility medications, both in terms of the number of follicles produced and the health of the eggs.

artificial insemination may be considered, but these patients are usually recommended to pursue IVF with intracytoplasmic sperm injection (ICSI).

Kristin comments:

Despite having a diagnosis of PCOS when I was referred to an RE, I still had to go through the regular battery of blood tests, ultrasounds, and an HSG. It was a really scary time because none of my friends had ever gone through any of the tests and I really felt like a pincushion. Besides the physical toll of the tests, it was definitely emotionally draining. I think the initial tests in some ways prepare you for the weeks of daily blood draws and ultrasounds that accompany IUI [intra-uterine insemination] and IVF. Before IVF I was terrified of needles, but within days I was a pro at giving myself shots.

9. What is ovarian reserve, and how is it tested?

Each month, during a woman's reproductive cycle, a single follicle is selected out of a group of potential follicles, reaches maturity, and ovulates a single egg. Many fertility treatments use medications to "rescue" other follicles from that group, so that multiple eggs are released during ovulation as opposed to just a single egg. If physicians could predict which patients would respond well to fertility treatments, then those women predicted to produce a low number of eggs with a poor chance of success with stimulated cycle IVF could defer this treatment and consider other options including unstimulated or Natural Cycle IVF (NC-IVF). Those women who respond well to fertility medications are described as having normal ovarian reserve. Those patients who have a poor response to fertility medications are described as having **diminished ovarian reserve**. Although patients with diminished ovarian reserve are likely to demonstrate suboptimal numbers of eggs during a stimulated IVF cycle, they may still conceive spontaneously, or with non-IVF treatments or with NC-IVF.

Ovarian reserve consists of two separate components, both of which determine a woman's chance of conceiving a child with IVF. The first component is the number of extra follicles that are available to undergo recruitment with treatment using fertility medications. This number depends on several factors, including the woman's chronological age (as discussed later), previous ovarian surgery, genetics, and exposure to environmental toxins (most notably, tobacco usage).

The second component is the actual health of the follicles and the eggs within those follicles. First and foremost, egg quality is determined by a woman's chronological age. Peak female fertility occurs when a woman is in her twenties and then drops significantly with age, especially following age 35. This fact has been conclusively demonstrated in many ways but is especially obvious when we look at IVF pregnancy rates. In patients who undergo IVF, studies have shown that around the age of 35 years old a marked decrease occurs in the chance of an embryo implanting successfully. In addition, the miscarriage rate rises with age, especially in those women older than age 40, in whom this rate exceeds 50%. Therefore, the age component of ovarian reserve is essentially immutable. In other words, unless she uses eggs from an egg donor, a woman cannot change her chronological age—and, with increasing age, the number of normal eggs inevitably falls sharply. Although it is true that the percentage of normal eggs within an ovary is specific to the individual woman, even the most fertile women possess very few normal eggs after age 40.

The concept of ovarian reserve testing, therefore, represents a means by which the physician attempts to evaluate a woman's reproductive potential both in terms of the number of follicles that remain and the health of those follicles. There are several ways in which one can assess ovarian reserve. First, follicle-stimulating hormone (FSH) can be measured on day 2 or 3 of a normal menstrual cycle. An estradiol level should be obtained at the same time, because the FSH level can be misleadingly low in women who have a high estrogen level early in the menstrual cycle. Alternatively, ovarian reserve can be assessed by performing a transvaginal ultrasound and counting the antral follicles present. In women with a slightly elevated FSH level, a transvaginal ultrasound may reveal a large number of follicles—somewhat reassuring the patient and her physician that perhaps her ovarian reserve is more normal than might otherwise be expected.

Unfortunately, normal FSH and estradiol levels do not guarantee a normal response to fertility medications. The **clomiphene citrate challenge test** (**CCCT**) was initially described as a means to identify those women with normal FSH and estradiol levels on day 3 of the menstrual cycle (**day-3 hormones**) who may demonstrate a suboptimal response to injectable fertility medications and poor IVF pregnancy rates. In the CCCT, the patient takes 100 mg of clomiphene citrate on cycle days 5 through 9. An FSH level is checked on days 3 and 10. If both of these levels are less than 10 IU/L (international units), then this represents a normal response. If the FSH level is greater than 10 IU/L on day 3 but less than 10 IU/L on day 10, then this represents a borderline situation, but is potentially reassuring based on the response of the ovary to stimulation with clomiphene citrate. If the FSH level is normal on day 3 but greater than 10 IU/L on day 10, however, the

Clomiphene citrate challenge test (CCCT)

A test used to evaluate a woman's ovarian reserve before she undergoes a fertility treatment.

Day-3 hormones

Measurement of follicle-stimulating hormone and estradiol on the second or third day of a regular menstrual cycle, which provides an assessment of a woman's ovarian reserve.

woman is likely to exhibit a suboptimal response to fertility medication, along with high IVF cancellation rates and poor pregnancy rates.

Antimullerian hormone (AMH) is another blood hormone test that is often used to assess ovarian reserve. Many experts believe that AMH is a better indicator of ovarian reserve than serum FSH as it has less cycle-to-cycle variability. See Question 10 for more information on AMH.

A word of caution is in order regarding ovarian reserve testing, including the CCCT: Virtually all physicians have patients who have successfully delivered a child following an abnormal CCCT. An abnormal CCCT or elevated FSH level on cycle day 3 does not preclude spontaneous pregnancy and delivery. Nevertheless, the miscarriage rate and the incidence of Down syndrome may be increased in such pregnancies. Patients with diminished ovarian reserve may have successful treatment with the combination of fertility drugs and intra-uterine insemination (IUI), or even with IUI alone. More recently, unstimulated or NC-IVF has gained increased popularity in treating patients with diminished ovarian reserve. A recent paper from Italy described 500 NC-IVF cycles in patients who had previously failed to respond to ovarian stimulation medications. In spite of having such a poor history, over 10% of the women under 40 years of age achieved a pregnancy. Considering that in the United States, most of these women would have been offered only donor egg IVF, we consider that pregnancy rate to be very remarkable.

The real benefit of ovarian reserve testing is its ability to identify often those patients in whom stimulated IVF is markedly less likely to be successful, allowing

The Fertility Evaluation and Treatment Basics

Antimullerian hormone (AMH)
A protein hormone that is used to evaluate a patient's ovarian reserve.

The real benefit of ovarian reserve testing is its ability to identify often those patients in whom stimulated IVF is markedly less likely to be successful.

23

Donor-egg IVF

An extremely successful type of in vitro fertilization procedure using the eggs from a young woman and with the resulting embryo(s) transferred into the recipient.

them to focus on other options such as NC-IVF, **donor-egg IVF**, adoption, or less invasive office-based fertility treatments. Overall, ovarian reserve testing represents an important factor when considering various fertility treatments and may be the final arbitrator in selecting the specific treatment plan.

Rebecca comments:

I first walked into my RE's office at the age of 39. I had just suffered the loss of a pregnancy that had taken me 8 months to conceive. I was very aware of the proverbial 'biological time clock' and was concerned that my husband and I may have run out of time. I was panic stricken about the tests that would evaluate my ovarian reserve; however, my desire to have children was greater than the fear I had about the test results. Fortunately, we found an RE who did not rely solely on my chronological age when he discussed our treatment options with us. He reviewed all my medical tests with me and offered an individualized plan that included a number of family building options that might address my infertility issues (most likely age related). Looking back, I realize how important our choice of RE was. It is important for women of advanced maternal age (AMA) to quickly identify an RE that is willing to work with, and is experienced in working with, women of AMA. An AMA woman must find a fertility clinic that offers a variety of fertility treatment options; one size (or one treatment) does NOT fit all. And finally, an AMA woman must find an RE who is willing to be aggressive in her treatment, but is also capable of being honest about the limitations of those treatment options for an AMA woman.

10. What is antimullerian hormone and what does this test tell my doctor?

AMH is a protein hormone produced by the cells that directly surround the egg, called the granulosa cells.

Granulosa cells (GC) also produce the hormones estrogen and progesterone. Since the cells that surround each egg produce AMH, we can measure a patient's blood AMH level and get a good determination of her total follicle pool or total egg count. If her AMH level is low, then her total follicle pool or egg count is also probably low. AMH offers additional insight into the patient's ovarian reserve in complementing other tests such as serum day 3 FSH, day 3 estradiol, clomiphene citrate challenge testing (CCCT), or ovarian "antral" follicle count (AFC) using ultrasonography. Since cycle day 3 FSH levels often fluctuate widely, a single measure of FSH may not represent a patient's true ovarian reserve especially if AMH and antral follicle count are normal.

The advantage of serum AMH testing is that AMH can be measured on any day of the patient's menstrual cycle. In other words, its levels are cycle day independent, so patients don't have to worry whether or not the blood sample is collected on day 3. Also, its levels tend to be more constant and more reliable for assessing ovarian reserve than day 3 serum FSH and estradiol. We often observe patients whose day 3 FSH and estradiol levels are normal, suggesting normal ovarian reserve, yet their AMH level is low and consistent with an observed low antral follicle count suggesting diminished ovarian reserve. Upon performing ovarian stimulation on such patients using **gonadotropins**, we often find that the AMH and antral follicle count properly identified the patient's true ovarian reserve better than using serum day 3 FSH and estradiol measurements.

At Dominion Fertility, we place much more emphasis on AMH levels than we do on the other blood markers for ovarian reserve. In Europe, AMH is also the preferred biomarker for assessing ovarian reserve in

Gonadotropins

Fertility medications containing follicle-stimulating hormone alone or in combination with luteinizing hormone.

25

many IVF centers but the use of AMH in the United States is becoming increasingly more popular.

11. What is a laparoscopy, and do I need one?

A laparoscopy is an outpatient surgery usually performed under general anesthesia. Most laparoscopies are completed in a hospital, but some physicians utilize freestanding outpatient surgery centers.

During a laparoscopy, the physician inserts a small fiber-optic telescope into the abdominal cavity through an incision made in the patient's umbilical area (belly button). Most physicians initially distend the abdomen using carbon dioxide gas with a needle (Veres needle) to create what is called a pneumoperitoneum. A trocar—an instrument with a diameter similar to that of a pencil—is then passed through the umbilicus, allowing for introduction of the telescope (called a laparoscope) into the abdomen.

Using the laparoscope, a gynecologic surgeon can inspect the uterus, fallopian tubes, and ovaries. The appendix and upper abdomen are carefully inspected as well. Additional instruments may be inserted into the abdomen through incisions (ports) made along the hairline above the pubic bone. For example, the physician may use graspers, scissors, or suction irrigators to rinse the tissue and remove blood and fluids as needed. Some physicians insert a slightly larger telescope through the umbilical port, which allows them to use a carbon dioxide laser to cut scar tissue or destroy implants of endometriosis. Besides the laser, other instruments can be used to cut or burn abnormalities such as endometriosis or scar tissue.

During a laparoscopy, the physician typically introduces a blue dye into the uterine cavity while directly visualizing the fallopian tubes. If the fallopian tubes are patent (open) but are located in an abnormal location because of scar tissue, then the surgeon may try to free the fallopian tubes to improve the patient's fertility.

If abnormal ovarian cysts such as endometriomas are present, then the physician may remove them during the course of the laparoscopy or, if necessary, perform a **laparotomy**. A laparotomy is a surgery performed through a larger incision, usually made along the bikini line. It may require the patient to stay 1 to 3 days in the hospital following the surgery. In addition, a laparotomy requires a longer recovery period and may create more new scar tissue than laparoscopic surgery.

Laparotomy
An inpatient surgical procedure that is performed through an open abdominal incision.

Certain abnormalities cannot be easily treated through laparoscopy, including exceedingly large ovarian cysts, ovarian cysts that are suspicious for cancer, and fibroids that are deeply embedded in the wall of the uterus. Patients with these problems are probably better served by a laparotomy.

For many years, all women who were seeking fertility care underwent laparoscopy as part of the initial evaluation. In recent times, this practice has faded with increased utilization of IVF. Although IVF has essentially replaced tubal surgery in patients with tubal factor infertility, laparoscopy is still used to correct certain problems in patients prior to undergoing IVF. For patients uninterested in IVF (for religious, financial or philosophical reasons), laparoscopy may still represent an important part of their diagnostic and therapeutic options. Complications of laparoscopy are rare but can include injury to the bowel, bladder, and blood vessels; a need for laparotomy; and even death.

12. What is a hysteroscopy, and do I need one? Is it the same as a water sonogram or a hysterosalpingogram?

A hysteroscopy is a simple surgical procedure that is performed either to diagnose or to treat a problem within the uterine cavity. During hysteroscopy, the physician inserts a small fiber-optic telescope through the cervix and into the uterus. Either gas or liquid can be used to distend the uterus and allow the physician to directly visualize the uterine cavity. The physician may also introduce small instruments into the uterus to cut scar tissue or remove polyps or fibroids. Although diagnostic hysteroscopy can be performed in the physician's office under local anesthesia, operative hysteroscopy usually requires anesthesia because of the cramping that occurs during uterine manipulation. Complications of hysteroscopy are rare but may include infection, bleeding, uterine perforation, damage to adjacent structures, and even death.

Hysterosonogram

A type of transvaginal sonogram performed after placement of a small catheter into the uterine cavity through which sterile water is introduced, allowing for visualization of the uterine cavity.

A water sonogram (**hysterosonogram**) is a specialized ultrasound examination performed using a transvaginal ultrasound probe. First, a small catheter is passed through the cervix and into the uterine cavity. Sterile saline is then introduced into the cavity while a transvaginal sonogram is performed, allowing the physician to visualize any uterine polyps or fibroids. Usually, a hysterosonogram does not provide any information about the status of the fallopian tubes. Nevertheless, hysterosonograms are helpful in identifying the presence of an endometrial polyp seen on routine sonogram or the location of a fibroid (see **Figure 3**). A hysterosonogram has limited benefit in evaluating for the presence of uterine scar tissue and is a diagnostic and not therapeutic procedure.

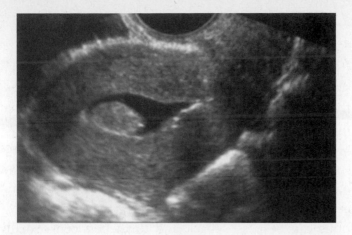

Figure 3   Sonohysterography showing a fibroid extending into the uterine cavity.

Source: © 2006 American Society for Reproductive Medicine.

A hysterosalpingogram (HSG) is similar to a hysterosonogram in that fluid is introduced into the uterine cavity. However, the fluid is not saline but rather is a radio-opaque dye. This dye is introduced into the uterus and, under fluoroscopy, the dye is observed as it sequentially fills the uterine cavity and then passes out into the fallopian tubes and ultimately spills out of the ends of the tubes and into the pelvis. The HSG can be used to diagnose polyps and fibroids and is superior to hysterosonogram in evaluating the presence of uterine scar tissue. This imaging procedure also provides information on the status of the fallopian tubes, unlike either a hysteroscopy or a hysterosonogram. Because it employs traditional x-rays, an HSG is usually performed at a hospital's radiology department or at a radiologist's office, since few REs have this equipment in their offices.

The Fertility Evaluation and Treatment Basics

13. What is ureaplasma, and how did I get it?

Most reproductive endocrinologists routinely obtain samples from the cervix (cervical cultures) to assess their patients for **gonorrhea**, **chlamydia**, **ureaplasma**, **mycoplasma**, and other bacterial infections. Gonorrhea and chlamydia are sexually-transmitted diseases that can cause tubal damage and infertility when these bacteria travel from the cervix through the uterus and out into the fallopian tubes. Sexually-transmitted infections can be passed back and forth between sexually intimate partners. Patients with gonorrhea may have a yellowish discharge associated with pelvic pain and fever. Although chlamydia can be associated with these symptoms, chlamydial infections are often silent. Despite their lack of symptoms, chlamydia infections may result in significant tubal scarring and damage.

Ureaplasma and mycoplasma are bacteria that can be commonly found in the reproductive tract of both men and women. It is somewhat more problematic to label these two bacteria as reproductive tract pathogens because they are often found in fertile, healthy couples in addition to those with infertility. Although the presence of these two bacteria has been hypothesized to play a role in both infertility and miscarriage, the specific mechanisms by which they impair fertility remains unclear. The question of whether ureaplasma or mycoplasma can cause reproductive tract damage or whether their presence increases the rate of miscarriage has not been definitively answered. As a consequence, many clinics do not test for ureaplasma or mycoplasma routinely.

If cervical cultures for ureaplasma and mycoplasma are positive, both the patient and her sexual partner are

Gonorrhea

A sexually transmitted disease that can cause tubal damage and infertility.

Chlamydia

A common sexually transmitted disease that can damage a woman's fallopian tubes.

Ureaplasma

A type of bacteria that may contribute to infertility.

Mycoplasma

A type of bacteria that may contribute to infertility.

usually treated with antibiotics such as doxycycline. As these bacteria may have been present for many years without causing any symptoms, the finding of ureaplasma and mycoplasma on cervical cultures does not in any way indicate infidelity or sexual misconduct.

14. Can infertility be unexplained?

The etiology (underlying cause) of infertility in many couples can be determined by various tests as previously described. Yet, there still remains a sizable percentage of couples in whom no obvious cause of infertility can be identified. Some studies estimate that approximately 10% to 20% of patients fall into this category. However, "unexplained infertility" is not necessarily equivalent to "untreatable infertility." If a couple has prolonged, unexplained infertility with no previous pregnancies, then a number of etiologies are possible.

If a woman is having normal, regular menstrual cycles, it is likely that each month a follicle is growing and that an egg is being released in an appropriate fashion. If pregnancy has never occurred, however, we cannot be sure that the woman's fallopian tubes are able to trap the egg or that her partner's sperm are able to swim through the cervix and uterus and find/fertilize the egg in the fallopian tube. In the absence of a previous pregnancy, the question arises as to whether fertilization can, in fact, occur. The scope of this problem is made clear when we look at the fertilization results for patients who undergo IVF with a diagnosis of unexplained infertility. Typically, the rate of failed fertilization with IVF is approximately 2%, but this rate increases dramatically—to approximately 20%—in couples who have prolonged unexplained infertility with no previous pregnancies. Ultimately, failed fertilization may result from problems with either sperm or egg, or both. In such cases of prolonged unexplained infertility, the use of intracytoplasmic sperm injection (ICSI) [see Question 53] can markedly reduce the rate of IVF fertilization failure since ICSI involves the direct injection of a single sperm into a mature egg. If a woman produces a sufficient number of eggs, then one option that we frequently employ is to split the eggs into two groups—ICSI and regular IVF. This split provides a control group, but if fertilization is poor without ICSI then IVF may ultimately prove to have been of diagnostic benefit.

One of the most significant developments in the treatment of infertile couples has been the move away from extensive diagnostic testing and toward a more rapid recommendation to undergo IVF. We often recommend that patients with prolonged unexplained infertility consider IVF with ICSI, as this combination has both diagnostic and therapeutic benefits.

Carol comments:

We were never able to diagnose the exact reason that I couldn't become pregnant. This can be frustrating and scary because there is no clear-cut path to fixing a problem that you can't define. I remember talking to other women who had more defined issues such as male factor or PCOS and thinking that those would be easier diagnoses to deal with. Luckily, we were able to benefit from the trend of REs to rapidly recommend IVF for patients whose infertility is unexplained.

15. After we have sex, I think that everything comes out. Is this why I am not getting pregnant?

Honestly, this question is one of the most frequently asked questions that we get during new patient consultations. At the time of male orgasm, the ejaculate is composed of proteins, enzymes, and water from the seminal vesicles. The sperm represent only one to three drops of the total ejaculate volume of 1.5 to 5 mL. Following ejaculation in the vagina sperm rapidly move from the vagina into the cervical mucus, where they can live for 5 to 7 days. The cervical mucus serves as a reservoir for the sperm, from which they can subsequently travel to the upper reproductive tract and meet the egg in the fallopian tube.

It is normal for much of the ejaculate to spill out of the vagina following coitus. For most couples, this does not decrease their chances for pregnancy. Rarely, a woman may suffer from vaginal or uterine prolapse. The altered anatomic relationship may not hold enough of the ejaculate in close proximity to the cervix following coitus. Such conditions usually occur only after several previous vaginal deliveries.

16. My friend keeps asking whether I had an endometrial biopsy or a postcoital test. Do I need these tests?

In the past, the **endometrial biopsy** was a routine part of the fertility evaluation, but currently it is performed mainly on patients at risk for endometrial cancer or with repeated IVF failures. An endometrial biopsy is a simple office-based procedure that is performed just before the onset of a woman's menses. It can be done without any anesthesia and is well-tolerated by most patients with the majority reporting uterine cramping that quickly resolves.

Endometrial biopsy

A sample of the lining of the uterus, usually performed to rule out endometrial cancer.

Although an endometrial biopsy can yield information about the hormonal status of the lining and can rule out chronic infection/inflammation in the uterus, its usefulness as a fertility test is limited by the fact that abnormal biopsies are obtained in more than one-third of women with proven fertility. Therefore, the finding of an abnormal endometrial biopsy in fertility patients is of uncertain benefit. Most reproductive endocrinologists prefer simply to have their patients take extra progesterone, essentially obviating the need for the endometrial biopsy in most patients. At the present time, the endometrial biopsy is most reliable as a means to rule out endometrial cancer in those patients who are at increased risk of this disease. Patients at increased risk for endometrial cancer include those who have polycystic ovarian syndrome and infrequent, heavy periods but who do not receive the protective benefit of oral contraceptives or other progesterone-containing medications.

In patients who have experienced repeated IVF failures in spite of the transfer of good quality embryos, it is reasonable to perform an endometrial biopsy to ensure that the lining demonstrates the appropriate hormonal response, the absence of infection/inflammation and even the correct expression of cell surface proteins called integrins that play a putative role in implantation. Abnormal integrin expression has been demonstrated in a range of clinical situations including the presence of a fluid filled fallopian tube or **hydrosalpinx**, but most experts consider testing for integrins to be investigational and limited to special circumstances.

The **postcoital test** was initially proposed as a means to evaluate the interaction of the male partner's sperm and the female partner's cervical mucus. This test is performed approximately 8 to 24 hours after intercourse at midcycle (around days 12 to 14 of the menstrual cycle). During a speculum exam, the physician collects a sample of cervical mucus. This sample is then placed on a slide and examined under a microscope for the presence of motile sperm. In addition to the presence or absence of

Hydrosalpinx

Obstruction of the fallopian tube at the fimbria, resulting in a fluid-filled and dilated tube.

Postcoital test

A test of historical interest used to assess the presence and behavior of sperm found within the cervical mucus.

sperm, the physician records the quality, quantity, and appearance of the mucus. Unfortunately, the postcoital test has very poor reproducibility and limited utility in the evaluation of infertile couples. For example, couples for whom no motile sperm were observed during the postcoital test have conceived. and although the spontaneous pregnancy rates are higher in those patients with a normal postcoital test, the information gathered in this way seldom provides any useful insight when developing a therapeutic plan.

Postcoital tests may prove more valuable in couples in whom, for social or religious reasons, the male partner is unable to provide a specimen for semen analysis. In these cases, a postcoital test reassures all parties that sperm are actually deposited in the vagina during the act of intercourse.

17. Can I choose the sex of my baby?

Gender is determined at the moment of fertilization, when a sperm bearing either an X or Y chromosome penetrates the egg, resulting in formation of either a female or male embryo, respectively. The event is random, and the sex ratio of females to males conceived is fairly even.

Several techniques exist that can enhance the likelihood that a couple will conceive a child with the desired gender. The Ericsson method is a simple, noninvasive method that separates X-bearing sperm from Y-bearing sperm using centrifugation techniques. The sperm are placed on the top of a column of either albumin or Sephadex, and the specimen is centrifuged to isolate the desired gender-selected sperm. This sperm sample is then used for either **intrauterine insemination** or IVF. The success rates reported with this method vary

The postcoital test has very poor reproducibility and limited utility in the evaluation of infertile couples.

Intrauterine insemination (IUI)

A fertility treatment in which the sperm are washed and then placed within the uterine cavity.

from no benefit to as high as 75% for the desired gender. The Ericsson method is not associated with any known risk to either baby or mother.

Microsort is a newer experimental technique that involves labeling the DNA of the sperm, followed by passage of the sample through a cell-sorting machine. This process yields a smaller sperm sample than the Ericsson method, and IVF with ICSI may be required for pregnancy. Nevertheless, the results appear encouraging in terms of gender selection.

The gender of a child can also be selected using IVF and preimplantation genetic diagnosis (PGD). This technique is expensive and much more complex than the Ericsson method, but success rates for the selected gender routinely exceed 90%. Couples who elect to pursue IVF and PGD for gender selection often do so to prevent genetically inheritable medical diseases, such as Duchenne muscular dystrophy, from occurring in their children.

Many medical authorities consider gender selection to be unethical except in a few circumstances, such as when the couple runs a high risk of having a child with an inheritable medical disease. Others support the use of gender selection when a couple has at least one child but wants to limit their family size and desires a child of the opposite gender.

18. How will my reproductive endocrinologist determine a plan of therapy?

In general, reproductive endocrinologists recommend a particular course of treatment only after performing a complete fertility evaluation that usually includes a pelvic ultrasound, an assessment of tubal patency

The Fertility Evaluation and Treatment Basics

(hysterosalpingogram or laparoscopy), a semen analysis, and a variety of hormonal blood tests.

The therapeutic plan for any couple is unique to them. If testing has demonstrated a clear problem, such as blocked fallopian tubes or a markedly abnormal sperm count, then in vitro fertilization (IVF) may be recommended as the only reasonable alternative. However, most couples are not sterile but merely subfertile, so they may be offered a range of therapeutic options—from expectant management, to the use of insemination with or without fertility drugs, to IVF with or without intracytoplasmic sperm injection (ICSI).

Most couples are not sterile but merely subfertile, so they may be offered a range of therapeutic options.

A couple's particular therapeutic plan should be developed with their specific needs in mind. For those patients in whom IVF is not an option, whether because of religious, financial, or philosophical reasons, the physician should provide counseling about alternative treatments available to them. Not all couples are prepared to undergo extensive fertility treatments, so physicians need to consider a couple's particular situation when proposing a course of action. Given that infertile couples can sometimes achieve spontaneous pregnancies, the desire of a couple to proceed with therapy needs to be weighed against the likelihood of success for that therapy and the cost involved. These costs may include financial, physical, and emotional considerations. We strongly urge our patients to consider all options when dealing with infertility, including alternative pathways to parenting ranging from adoption to the use of donor sperm, donor egg, donor embryo, and gestational surrogacy.

Carol comments:

I feel that finding an RE who will work with you and listen to you is one of the most important factors in achieving a positive outcome. Each individual who is faced with infertility deals with the varying costs (financial, physical, and emotional) differently. For some, the financial aspect limits the number of attempts they can make. For others, the physical and emotional aspects take such a toll that they are only willing to go through a set number of attempts. Based on my discussions with other women who have faced fertility challenges, I believe that each person has a unique threshold for these costs. If you are dealing with a doctor who strictly adheres to a "one size fits all" policy and won't take your personal situation into consideration, it will only add more stress to an already stressful situation.

19. What are natural cycle fertility treatments and am I a candidate for them?

Natural cycle fertility treatments are based entirely on a woman's normal natural menstrual cycle. In other words, no ovarian stimulating drugs are used. Rather, the doctor attempts to achieve a pregnancy using the woman's naturally produced egg and/or hormones. In order to use any form of natural fertility treatment, the patient must have fairly regular menstrual cycles. Highly irregular cycles do not allow the use of natural fertility treatment. Three different types of natural fertility treatments currently exist and they are Natural Cycle IUI, Natural Cycle IVF, and Natural Cycle FET.

Natural Cycle IUI

Natural Cycle IUI is an extremely simple infertility treatment. Generally speaking, the patient is monitored during a menstrual cycle to determine the timing of ovulation using either urine LH, blood estradiol and progesterone or sonography. Once the egg has been determined to be mature, ovulation can be induced by a single injection of **human chorionic gonadotropin (HCG)** followed by a well-timed artificial insemination

Human chorionic gonadotropin (HCG)

A placental hormone produced in pregnancy that is the basis for blood and urine pregnancy testing.

(IUI). Sometimes IUI is performed without the use of HCG if it appears that an LH surge has already begun based upon hormone testing. See Questions 37–44 for more information about IUI.

Natural Cycle IVF (NC-IVF)

Natural Cycle IVF (NC-IVF) also requires that the patient have regular menstrual cycles. NC-IVF is a very simple, patient-friendly form of IVF. No ovarian stimulating drugs are used in NC-IVF. Instead, the patient's naturally produced follicle and egg are monitored using estradiol, progesterone and ultrasound measurements. Once the egg is judged to be mature, a single injection of HCG is given and the egg is easily collected in the office under transvaginal ultrasound using minimal or no sedation. It literally takes only a few minutes to collect the egg, similar to a simple in-office blood draw. The egg is then fertilized, usually by ICSI (as only one egg is obtained), and a single embryo is transferred 3 or 5 days later. Couples with proven previous fertility may use IVF without ICSI in many cases.

NC-IVF is extensively performed around the world in more than 50 countries and the world's very first successful IVF baby was produced in 1978, using NC-IVF. At that time, our knowledge and technology were rudimentary compared with today's standards, so fertility drugs were ultimately used to obtain more eggs and embryos to improve the very low IVF pregnancy rates. With improved understanding and technology, many eggs and embryos are simply not necessary to produce a successful pregnancy for many couples using IVF. Also the costs for NC-IVF are about 20%–25% of the cost of a single stimulated IVF cycle and NC-IVF avoids the risks associated with the use of ovarian stimulating hormones. Thus, patients who are planning

The Fertility Evaluation and Treatment Basics

on a single embryo transfer or who wish to avoid using fertility drugs often prefer NC-IVF. Patients who fail stimulated IVF or who wish to try NC-IVF with their own egg prior to considering ova donor IVF may be candidates for NC-IVF.

Problems with NC-IVF include: premature LH surge, which occurs in 10%–15% of patients and, less commonly, failure to obtain an egg at the time of the follicle aspiration. Occasionally, fertilization may not occur (even with the use of ICSI) or embryo growth may be suboptimal with failure of an embryo to develop to an appropriate stage prior to planned embryo transfer. When compared with stimulated IVF utilizing single embryo transfer, the pregnancy rates should be similar between NC-IVF and stimulated IVF. Studies comparing these two types of IVF are needed but our personal experience supports this notion. For more on NC-IVF see Question 59.

Natural Cycle Frozen Embryo Transfer (NC-FET)

Frozen embryo transfer (FET)

Placement of previously cryopreserved embryos into the uterus or, more rarely, the fallopian tube.

A **frozen embryo transfer** cycle involves the placement of embryo from what were cryopreserved in a prior IVF cycle into the uterus. The lining of the uterus must be ready for the embryos to implant and the timing of embryo transfer is understandably very important. NC-FET can be offered to patients who have regular menstrual cycles. NC-FET is less expensive, simpler for the patient and the pregnancy rates are equal to medicated FET. During NC-FET, the menstrual cycle is monitored in the same fashion as previously described for NC-IUI and NC-IVF. A single injection (HCG) is given to the patient to induce ovulation and provide correct timing for the embryo transfer 7 days later. It's just that simple! The entire treatment takes one menstrual cycle or about 4 weeks to complete.

We have been performing NC-FET for several years now and our data shows equal pregnancy rates with NC-FET or medicated FET. In our opinion, the only drawback to NC-FET is that it requires the IVF center and patient to be flexible with respect to scheduling of the embryo transfer as this date can only be estimated at the start of the cycle. With a medicated FET, the exact date and time of the embryo transfer can be programmed before beginning the treatment. For more about NC-FET and medicated FET see Questions 71–73.

20. How expensive are infertility treatments?

Some insurance plans may cover the cost of a fertility evaluation but not cover any fertility treatments per se. Other plans may stipulate a certain lifetime benefit for fertility cases and still other plans may provide a specific number of treatment cycles.

For patients without insurance coverage, the cost of fertility treatments varies widely depending on the specific treatment utilized. For example, in many clinics, a cycle of ultrasound monitoring without the use of fertility medications, culminating with intrauterine insemination (IUI), may cost $1,300 to $1,500. Compare this with the cost of IVF with intracytoplasmic sperm injection, freezing of extra embryos, and assisted embryo hatching, for which the price tag can total $14,000 to $16,000 (not including the cost of injectable fertility medications [$2,000 to $4,000]). The use of donor-egg IVF, although extremely successful, is also very expensive, because the donor must be reimbursed for her time and effort as part of the treatment and also because of the extensive screening tests mandated by the FDA. The price for donor-egg IVF typically ranges between

Some insurance plans may cover the cost of a fertility evaluation but not cover any fertility treatments per se.

$25,000 and $30,000, depending on the clinic. Unstimulated or Natural Cycle IVF may represent an economically attractive, albeit less successful, option since it costs a fraction of stimulated cycle IVF (e.g. $4,400 per cycle in our clinic).

For most patients, the more expensive, more invasive fertility treatments usually result in the highest pregnancy rates. Couples are advised to carefully consider the proposed course of treatment and the costs that may be involved.

Many IVF centers in the United States offer "money back" (refund) programs. A couple accepted into such a program pays a premium that covers several fresh IVF cycles as well as frozen embryo transfers (FET). If they fail to conceive or are deemed to no longer be appropriate candidates for treatment, then all or a percentage of their initial payment is refunded. These programs have remained somewhat controversial but can allow couples to pursue other options if IVF proves unsuccessful.

According to the ASRM Ethics Committee Statement of June 2006, the controversy surrounding such programs relates in part to the concern that such arrangements appear to violate long-standing ethical prohibitions against paying contingency fees in medicine. This concern is based on Opinion 6.01 of the AMA Code of Medical Ethics, which states, "a physician's fee should not be made contingent on the successful outcome of a medical treatment."

Furthermore, the 2006 Committee Statement (which can be found on the ASRM website at http://www. asrm.org/Media/Ethics/ethicsmain.html) concludes, "the risk-sharing form of payment for IVF is an option that might be ethically offered to patients without health insurance coverage for IVF if certain conditions that protect patient interests are met. These conditions are that the criterion of success is clearly specified, that patients are fully informed of the financial costs and advantages and disadvantages of such programs, that informed consent materials clearly inform patients of their chances of success if found eligible for the risk-sharing program, and that the program is not guaranteeing pregnancy and delivery. It should also be clear to patients that they will be paying a higher cost for IVF if they do, in fact, succeed on the first or second cycle than if they had not chosen the risk-sharing program, and that, in any event, the costs of screening and drugs are not included.

"The Committee was especially concerned about the incentives that risk-sharing programs create for providers to take actions that might harm patients in order to achieve success and avoid a refund. For risk-sharing programs to be ethical, it is imperative that patients be aware of this potential conflict of interest and that risk-sharing programs not overstimulate patients to obtain a large supply of eggs or transfer more embryos than is safe for the patient, fetus, and prospective offspring. Patients should be fully informed of the risks of multifetal gestation for mother and fetus, and have ample time to discuss and consider them prior to egg retrieval."

21. Will my insurance pay for my fertility treatments?

Insurance coverage for infertility varies widely across the United States. Several states, including Massachusetts, Illinois, and Maryland, have passed legislative mandates for infertility coverage. In these states, access to fertility treatment is guaranteed through the patient's employer. In the vast majority of states, however, fertility coverage is inconsistent. Some companies may offer extensive fertility benefits, while others offer no coverage at all to their employees.

It is important that you understand your specific benefits before you seek out any kind of fertility treatment. Insurance plans may provide a specific dollar amount to spend on fertility treatments or cover a certain number of cycles of either IUI or IVF. You should work with your fertility provider's billing staff to determine which benefits are available to you before launching into a treatment plan. Given that some insurance plans may cover infertility more extensively than others, it is always appropriate to examine your insurance options during periods of open enrollment for health benefits. Many insurance companies will not cover fertility treatments in patients who have been voluntarily sterilized (e.g., **vasectomy, tubal ligation**). Plans may also have specific requirements in terms of duration of fertility and exclusion criteria for IVF concerning ovarian reserve testing or age.

Rebecca comments:

One of the biggest mistakes I made in my family building journey was making 'assumptions' about my husband's and my insurance plans. These assumptions, NOT FACTS, guided some of our initial decision making processes regarding treatment. Those errors in judgment wasted precious time, and most likely were financially costly. As a wiser and more seasoned patient, I would advise that one take as much precaution and care in learning about her/his insurance coverage, as one does with obtaining information about her/his treatment options. Work with the fertility provider's billing staff regarding your plan and benefits as soon as you begin consulting with your RE.

Vasectomy
Surgical sterilization of a man by cutting the vas deferens.

Tubal ligation
Surgical sterilization of a woman, performed by cutting or occluding the fallopian tubes.

PART THREE

Specific Problems: Polycystic Ovarian Syndrome (PCOS)

Why are my menstrual cycles irregular?

What is polycystic ovarian syndrome? Where does it come from and how is it treated?

I have PCOS and am still not having normal cycles with metformin. What comes next?

More ...

22. Why are my menstrual cycles irregular?

In a typical reproductive cycle, a single follicle (containing a single egg) reaches maturity after 2 weeks, culminating with the release of that egg in a process called ovulation. Once ovulation has occurred, a menstrual period will occur 12-14 days later unless pregnancy supervenes. Thus, most women cycle every 28 days (14 days to grow the egg and 14 days after ovulation until period returns).

If a woman has irregular and unpredictable cycles, then logic suggests that she is probably not ovulating normally.

Understandably, if a woman has irregular and unpredictable cycles, then logic suggests that she is probably not ovulating normally. Ovulatory problems are usually divided into two main categories: problems with the ovary and problems with the signals from the brain to the ovary. If the irregular cycles result from a lack of follicles within her ovary, then the failure of the ovary to respond will cause the pituitary gland to secrete increased amounts of follicle-stimulating hormone (FSH). Women with elevated levels of FSH are described as having diminished ovarian reserve; if their periods cease entirely, then they are described as having **premature ovarian failure (POF)**. Laboratories may differ as to how they define an "elevated" level of FSH, so a discussion with your physician is crucial to correctly assess the results of this test. In most cases, however, an FSH level of more than 15 IU/L is evidence of diminished ovarian reserve; FSH levels exceeding 30 IU/L usually signify POF.

Premature ovarian failure (POF)

Irregular or absent menstrual cycles before the age of 40 years old, resulting from a marked loss of ovarian follicles as evidenced by a high blood level of follicle-stimulating hormone (FSH > 30 IU).

If a woman has a normal complement of follicles but still does not have normal cycles, then the problem must lie elsewhere. Most such women suffer from a communication mismatch between the brain and ovary, disrupting the carefully coordinated hormone signals that induce the growth of ovarian follicles. The causes of this disruption can be further classified, with most patients being found to have polycystic ovarian syndrome (see Question 23) as opposed to other hormonal imbalances.

23. What is polycystic ovarian syndrome? Where does it come from and how is it treated?

Polycystic ovarian syndrome (PCOS) is an exceedingly common reproductive disorder, affecting an estimated 10% to 15% of reproductive-age women. The diagnosis of PCOS is a clinical one. In 2003, the ESHRE/ASRM consensus conference redefined PCOS as the presence of at least two out of the three following clinical criteria:

1. Irregular menstrual cycles
2. Evidence of extra male hormones, as determined either by clinical examination or by blood tests
3. Ultrasound demonstrating ovaries with numerous small follicles (PCO-appearing ovaries)

Previously, only patients with irregular menstrual cycles were thought to have PCOS, so the expansion of this definition has led to some confusion among healthcare providers. Other features commonly associated with PCOS include obesity, **insulin resistance**, borderline diabetes, skin tags, and a velvety discoloration on the nape of the neck and inner thighs called **acanthosis nigricans**. The topic of PCOS can fill an entire book. In fact, several books have been devoted to this subject. Although this condition was originally described by Drs. Stein and Leventhal in 1935, our understanding of PCOS has advanced significantly in the last decade.

Originally, PCOS was thought to be an anatomical problem in which a thickened coating around the ovary

Insulin resistance

Impaired response to insulin, which can lead eventually to diabetes.

Acanthosis nigricans

A velvety skin discoloration associated with insulin resistance.

PCOS
*represents a
hormonal
imbalance.*

prevented ovulation. It is now agreed that PCOS represents a hormonal imbalance. At the heart of this disorder is insulin resistance. Insulin is a hormone secreted by the pancreas and induces your body to store the sugar circulating in the bloodstream. Individuals who fail to produce insulin as a result of an autoimmune disorder require insulin therapy to maintain normal blood sugar levels. These patients are referred to as having insulin-dependent diabetes (also known as type 1 diabetes).

The majority of patients with impaired glucose metabolism actually suffer from insulin resistance rather than insulin deficiency. That is, the cells of their bodies are not sensitive to the effects of insulin, so they require ever-increasing amounts of insulin to be released from the pancreas until appropriate blood levels of glucose are obtained. These patients are commonly referred to as having non-insulin-dependent diabetes (also known as type 2 diabetes or adult-onset diabetes). Despite the name of the disease, persons with type 2 diabetes may require insulin injections to maintain normal glucose levels depending on their degree of insulin resistance.

Insulin resistance is likely a genetic disorder. This explains why adult-onset type 2 diabetes is so prevalent in certain families and in certain ethnic groups. In patients who are insulin resistant, the excessive levels of insulin affect not only their metabolism, but also their reproductive system. Insulin directly affects the release of reproductive hormones from the pituitary gland and directly stimulates ovarian production of male hormones. Thus the presence of excess insulin results in a local environment that is not conducive to follicle growth. The multiple follicles that fail to mature produce excessive male hormones, resulting in acne and abnormal hair growth commonly encountered in women with PCOS. Obesity itself also increases insulin resistance, so patients can find themselves trapped in a vicious cycle of irregular cycles and worsening weight gain. Women who have always had regular periods during their entire life but suddenly gain significant weight may frequently resemble patients with PCOS. In these cases, weight loss by itself may restore normal cycles and improve fertility.

Kristin comments:

Looking back at my early menstrual cycles, it should have come as no surprise that my reproductive system was not in normal working order. I had extremely heavy periods, but they were never regular. Sometimes I would go months without a period. I didn't think much about it until my husband and I started trying to get pregnant. I went off the pill and got a period about 2 months later. I began charting my basal body temperature and discovered that I was not ovulating. I decided to be proactive and saw my OB, who confirmed that I have PCOS. This diagnosis was further confirmed at my first RE visit. The doctor did a transvaginal ultrasound, which showed that both of my ovaries were covered with many small follicles. I did meet the clinical criteria for diagnosing PCOS, but I did not exhibit any of the outwardly apparent features—obesity, skin tags, acanthosis nigricans.

Weight loss by itself may restore normal cycles and improve fertility.

24. If I have PCOS, why do I need to take metformin? Isn't that a drug for diabetics?

The role of insulin resistance as the probable initiating factor in PCOS has important clinical implications. Because of the pioneering work done by Drs. John Nestler and Andrea Dunaif, the treatment of patients with PCOS has now shifted toward addressing the underlying issue of insulin resistance. Patients with PCOS are often treated with an insulin-sensitizing medication such as metformin (Glucophage). More than 20% of patients with PCOS and irregular cycles will experience a restoration of their normal cycles with metformin treatment. Because most patients who take metformin experience a diminished appetite, they may also benefit from weight loss with this therapy. Patients with PCOS also have increased rates of first-trimester miscarriage, and preliminary data suggest that there is a reduced rate of miscarriage in patients with PCOS who are treated with metformin.

In order to minimize the gastrointestinal side effects, the dose of metformin is increased gradually. Many physicians initially prescribe 500 mg a day of the extended-release preparation of metformin, to be taken at dinner. After 1 week, the dose is increased to 1,000 mg; after another week, the dose is increased to the maximum of 1,500 mg. Most patients can tolerate the medication, although severe gastrointestinal side effects (mainly diarrhea) arise in 10% to 15% of patients. Patients who fail to resume predictable cycles with metformin therapy alone will need to consider ovulation induction with fertility medications.

Patients who fail to resume predictable cycles with metformin therapy alone will need to consider ovulation induction with fertility medications.

The use of metformin as a first-line medication in the treatment of ovulation problems in patients with PCOS is controversial. Some physicians believe that clomiphene should be the first medication prescribed to women with PCOS who desire pregnancy and have irregular cycles. Our preference has been to start with metformin and then add clomiphene if a women fails to resume regular menstrual cycles.

Kristin comments:

My OB suggested I try metformin to regulate my cycles. I started on 500 mg and eventually went up to 1,000 mg—and it worked. I started to get regular periods. By charting my basal body temperature, I could tell that I was ovulating. I experienced major gastrointestinal issues with the drug, but they subsided after a month or so with some flare-ups on occasion. The side effects were worth it as far as I was concerned, especially if the metformin was going to help me get pregnant. When I started seeing an RE, my metformin dose was upped to 1,500 mg. Once I did get pregnant through IVF, I remained on metformin for the first trimester of my pregnancy.

25. I have PCOS and am still not having normal cycles with metformin. What comes next?

In our experience, most patients who will resume regular cycles on metformin will demonstrate regular cycles within 4 months of starting this medication. Patients who fail to respond to metformin may require ovulation induction with either clomiphene citrate (Clomid) or injectable fertility medications (gonadotropins).

Clomid has been an FDA-approved treatment for **anovulation** since the late 1960s. This anti-estrogen has been used successfully in millions of women with few complications. Clomid binds to estrogen receptors in the brain, causing the pituitary gland to resume normal release of FSH, and thereby inducing follicles to grow and ultimately release an egg. Patients should take the lowest effective dose of Clomid needed to induce ovulation. With increasing doses, the anti-estrogen side effects can reduce fertility by altering the cervical mucus and leading to a thinner endometrial lining. Many physicians initially prescribe a dose of 50 mg of Clomid to be taken on cycle days 5 to 9. The physician may

Anovulation

Failure to release an egg on a regular basis, resulting in irregular or absent periods.

perform ultrasound monitoring after day 12. Most patients will ovulate around day 17. If no dominant follicle emerges by this day, then an increased dose of 100 mg should be considered in the next cycle. A dose of 150 mg is rarely prescribed, because the vast majority of Clomid-responsive patients will ovulate while taking the 50- or 100-mg dose. Patients who ovulate rarely or not at all can be given medroxyprogesterone acetate (Provera) for 10 days to induce bleeding. By convention, the first day of this bleeding is referred to as cycle day #1 (even though it was an induced bleed and not the result of a normal cycle) and clomiphene is prescribed as previously noted.

Women with PCOS who fail to respond to Clomid can be treated with injectable fertility hormones called gonadotropins.

Ovarian hyperstimulation syndrome (OHSS)

Ovarian enlargement, abdominal fluid retention, and dehydration following the use of fertility medication to induce the growth of multiple follicles.

Women with PCOS who fail to respond to Clomid can be treated with injectable fertility hormones called gonadotropins. Such hormone medications are prepared using either recombinant DNA technology (Follistim, Gonal-F) or by isolating these hormones from the urine of postmenopausal women (Bravelle, Menopur). By following a very-low-dose protocol (37.5 IU as the starting dose), approximately 90% of patients will achieve a single dominant follicle. If the treatment produces multiple follicles, however, the woman's risk of multiple pregnancy and **ovarian hyperstimulation syndrome (OHSS)** may lead to cycle cancellation. Alternatives to canceling the cycle and withholding HCG include conversion to IVF or performing a follicle aspiration procedure to reduce the number of follicles to a reasonable number but without fertilizing the eggs that were removed by the aspiration procedure. Almost all of the high-order multiple pregnancies (e.g., sextuplets) born today result from PCOS patients who took gonadotropins and demonstrated an excessive follicular response (think Jon and Kate Plus Eight).

26. If I don't have either PCOS or POF, then what is my problem and why am I not ovulating?

Hormone abnormalities other than PCOS can also lead to irregular menstrual cycles. Such abnormalities include problems with the thyroid gland (which produces a hormone that controls metabolism), abnormal levels of prolactin (a hormone that induces breast milk production), and a lack of hypothalamic/pituitary stimulation to the ovary known as **functional hypothalamic amenorrhea (FHA)**. The pituitary gland has been called the master gland of the body; it secretes hormones that control a wide range of functions, including reproduction, metabolism, response to stress, water balance, and growth.

Women with irregular cycles should have both their thyroid hormone and prolactin levels measured, as problems with the thyroid gland can indirectly lead to elevations in prolactin. Low levels of thyroid hormone (hypothyroidism) and elevations in prolactin (**hyperprolactinemia**) can be readily treated with medication. In fact, treatment of hypothyroidism with oral thyroid hormone (levothyroxine) can promptly restore normal menstruation. Similarly, hyperprolactinemia usually responds quickly to bromocriptine therapy, often promptly restoring normal cycles.

An elevation of prolactin in the absence of any thyroid disease requires magnetic resonance imaging (MRI) of the brain to evaluate its cause. In such cases, hyperprolactinemia usually results from an increased growth of the prolactin-secreting cells in the pituitary gland forming a small tumor. If the prolactin-secreting tumor is less than 1 cm in diameter, then it is called a **microadenoma**,

Functional hypothalamic amenorrhea (FHA)

The absence of menstrual cycles related to failure of the hypothalamus and pituitary gland to stimulate follicular growth.

Hyperprolactinemia

Excessive secretion of the hormone prolactin.

Microadenoma

A tumor of the pituitary gland measuring less than 1 cm.

Macroadenoma

A tumor of the pituitary gland measuring more than 1 cm.

whereas a **macroadenoma** is greater than 1 cm in diameter. These are not life-threatening conditions and usually respond very well to medication, which is well tolerated with few side effects.

Women without thyroid or prolactin issues, and with low or normal FSH levels, who fail to have menstrual periods following treatment with progesterone are usually referred to as having functional hypothalamic amenorrhea (FHA). These women demonstrate no follicle growth and therefore fail to produce normal levels of estrogen despite an appropriate complement of ovarian follicles. Women who are below ideal body weight and who exercise frequently and vigorously are particularly prone to developing this problem. Women with FHA are at risk for **osteoporosis** and should discuss with their physician the benefits of hormone therapy (such as oral contraceptives) when not attempting pregnancy. They should also undergo an MRI of the brain to rule out any structural etiology for their condition. Women who are below ideal body weight may resume normal menstrual cycles when they gain weight or decrease their exercise frequency and duration.

Osteoporosis

Loss of calcium and bone mass, leading to an increased risk of fracture.

Infertility in women with FHA can be readily treated with injectable gonadotropins. In such women, the choice of medication is important as the drug should contain both FSH and LH (Menopur) and not just FSH alone (Gonal-F, Follistim). Clomid rarely works in women with FHA, but nearly all women with FHA can undergo successful ovulation induction. As was discussed in the preceding question, an excessive response may lead to high order multiple pregnancy, so care should be taken to cancel such a cycle or convert it to IVF or consider a follicle reduction procedure.

PART FOUR

Specific Problems: Tubal Disease

Can fallopian tubes be repaired and why would a blocked tube be an issue if I am doing IVF anyway?

If I had my tubes tied, can I have them untied?

If I had a previous ectopic pregnancy, what should I do to avoid another one?

27. Can fallopian tubes be repaired and why would a blocked tube be an issue if I am doing IVF anyway?

Prior to the advent of IVF, surgical repair of damaged fallopian tubes was considered standard medical care. Unfortunately, most patients did not become pregnant following this procedure, and 10% to 20% experienced tubal (ectopic) pregnancies. Today, IVF has replaced reparative tubal surgery for most patients with damaged fallopian tubes for two reasons: (1) IVF is a nonsurgical treatment, and (2) it results in excellent pregnancy rates, especially for patients with tubal disease.

Some patients ask, "Why is it so difficult to repair damaged tubes?" Unfortunately, the problems that cause tubal disease, such as pelvic infections, usually damage the tubal **fimbria**—the delicate finger-like projections at the end of the tube that are responsible for capturing the egg when it is released from the ovary. Pelvic infections may also damage the entire thickness of the tube from the tubal muscle to the inner mucosal layer, leaving behind a scarred, nonfunctional organ that is not amenable to surgical repair.

Fimbria

The finger-like projections at the distal end of the fallopian tube that are responsible for trapping the egg following ovulation.

Most patients with tubal disease are best treated using IVF.

In general, most patients with tubal disease are best treated using IVF. Tubal reparative surgery is usually not effective and, in fact, it may increase the woman's risk for having an ectopic or tubal pregnancy. If a couple is not interested in IVF or if they are not deemed to be good candidates for IVF, then tubal surgery may be the only option available to them in terms of fertility treatment.

Damage to the fimbria of the fallopian tubes may result in a tube that is blocked at the very distal end—the part farthest away from the uterus. A tube that becomes filled with fluid is called a hydrosalpinx ("hydro" refers to water; "salpinx" refers to the fallopian tube itself). A hydrosalpinx is usually discovered during a hysterosalpingogram (HSG) performed as part of the infertility diagnostic evaluation. This simple x-ray study should be performed in all infertile women (unless a diagnostic laparoscopy has already been performed) as assessment of the status of the fallopian tubes is a key part of the fertility evaluation. We advise all patients undergoing a laparoscopy that we recommend removal or ligation of her tube(s) if a hydrosalpinx is discovered.

Over the past decade, many studies have demonstrated reduced IVF pregnancy rates in patients who have a hydrosalpinx. It has been theorized that the fluid in the tube may flow backward into the uterine cavity. This fluid may contain toxic substances that may adversely affect the receptivity of the endometrium, preventing implantation. Alternatively, the fluid may actually flush the embryo out of the cavity or even prove toxic to the embryo itself. Some studies suggest that the presence of an untreated hydrosalpinx will reduce IVF pregnancy rates by 50%. In addition, an untreated hydrosalpinx may increase the chance that a woman will experience a spontaneous abortion or miscarriage. For all these reasons, treating a hydrosalpinx should both increase the IVF pregnancy rate and decrease the chances for an early pregnancy loss. A patient with a single normal fallopian tube and a hydrosalpinx will also have a higher chance of achieving a spontaneous pregnancy after removal or ligation of the damaged tube.

28. If I had my tubes tied, can I have them untied?

Fertile women who have had their "tubes tied" (tubal ligation) may do very well and achieve pregnancy with tubal reanastomosis surgery. Pregnancy rates of 70% to 80% are noted in women who undergo a tubal reversal procedure, depending on their age, the type of tubal ligation procedure performed, and the presence (or absence) of other infertility factors.

Most often, this repair (**tubal reanastamosis**) requires a laparotomy, which involves a bikini-line incision of the lower abdomen. This major surgery requires 2 to 4 weeks for recovery, and most insurers do not cover it. Some physicians have reported good success with laparoscopic tubal reanastamosis, but this approach can be more technically challenging. As a consequence, most women choose to undergo a nonsurgical IVF procedure instead. Studies have shown that IVF is usually more cost-effective than surgical reanastomosis of the fallopian tubes. Specifically, if the surgery fails to establish a pregnancy, then IVF may be necessary anyway. Patients with a previous tubal ligation are usually excellent candidates for IVF, including Natural Cycle or unstimulated IVF, given their previous fertility.

However, patients who are shown to have diminished ovarian reserve with a history of a previous tubal ligation should be carefully advised of the potential for a poor response to fertility medications. In such cases, tubal reanastamosis or Natural Cycle IVF may represent more appropriate options.

Women who have experienced an ectopic pregnancy generally have a 10% to 15% risk for another ectopic pregnancy.

29. If I had a previous ectopic pregnancy, what should I do to avoid another one?

The reported incidence of tubal or ectopic pregnancy in the general population is 1%. Women who have experienced an ectopic pregnancy generally have a 10% to 15% risk for another ectopic pregnancy. The good news is that most women who have had an ectopic pregnancy will not have another one. The bad news is there are no options available to eliminate this risk entirely except adoption. All women who are attempting to conceive are inherently at risk for an ectopic pregnancy. Even women with absent or obstructed fallopian tubes can experience an ectopic pregnancy with IVF if the embryo becomes implanted in the section of the fallopian tube found within the muscle of the uterus (called an interstitial or cornual pregnancy). The rate of ectopic pregnancy following IVF is usually 1% to 2%, far lower than the 15% recurrence risk with a spontaneous pregnancy.

Fortunately, most ectopic pregnancies are readily diagnosed very early in pregnancy using blood hormone assays for beta human chorionic gonadotropin (HCG) combined with transvaginal ultrasonography. It is now uncommon for such pregnancies to go undiagnosed leading to tubal rupture, hemorrhage, or death. Most ectopic pregnancies can be treated medically using low doses of methotrexate (a type of chemotherapy that selectively destroys the pregnancy tissue), thereby avoiding surgery. This medical therapy is 80% to 95% effective.

Kristin comments:

I had an ectopic pregnancy after a Clomid cycle that was monitored by my OB. I was 8 to 9 weeks pregnant and thought I was having a miscarriage when the ectopic pregnancy was confirmed at my first RE appointment. Unfortunately, the methotrexate therapy did not work, and I had to have surgery to remove my right fallopian tube. After determining that my remaining tube was not blocked through an HSG, and with the counsel of our new RE, we opted to move on to IVF. This option would offer the greatest chance for us to become pregnant and avoid another ectopic pregnancy.

When I did become pregnant through IVF, my RE agreed to a very early ultrasound to make sure that the pregnancy was in my uterus. I appreciated that my RE understood my concerns of having another ectopic pregnancy. He treated me as an individual instead of requiring me to wait until the typical 7-week mark to perform an ultrasound.

PART FIVE

Specific Problems: Male Factors

Is there anything my husband can do to improve his sperm count, such as wearing boxers and not briefs, taking vitamins or undergoing surgery?

Should I consider using a sperm donor to conceive?

More . . .

30. Is there anything my husband can do to improve his sperm count, such as wearing boxers and not briefs, taking vitamins or undergoing surgery?

Semen analysis results demonstrate considerable variation from sample to sample, which complicates research efforts to identify specific dietary or lifestyle change that might potentially improve sperm quality. Although the presence of a **varicocele** has been suggested to play a role in male infertility, the benefit of **varicocelectomy** remains controversial.

Some studies have suggested that wearing boxers instead of briefs can improve a man's sperm count. The avoidance of extremely high temperature may also improve sperm counts, so care should be taken to avoid prolonged exposure to extremely high temperatures, such as within a sauna or a hot tub. Years ago on Long Island, Dr. Gordon had a patient whose husband owned a pizzeria. Once he stopped working 18 hours a day in front of the pizza ovens and moved to the cash register and away from the heat, his sperm count normalized and they conceived spontaneously.

The effects of a variety of nutritional supplements on semen have been studied with some researchers suggesting that antioxidants may improve sperm quality, thereby leading to improved pregnancy rates (the desired outcome). Although the data on nutritional supplements with antioxidant properties are somewhat limited, a commercially available product based on this research is available (Proceed, Sigma-Tau Pharmaceuticals). This nutritional supplement is available for purchase only over the Internet. Although it has been frequently prescribed by some urologists, additional studies are required to confirm its benefits.

Varicocele

One or more dilated veins often located in the scrotal sac and thought to be a possible cause of male infertility.

Varicocelectomy

Ligation of dilated testicular or inguinal veins thought to be a source of male infertility.

Surgical treatments for male factor infertility are very limited. Historically, varicocelectomy has been the surgical procedure most commonly used to improve sperm quality. In this procedure, dilated veins in the scrotum (varicocele) are cut or occluded. One theory is that these dilated veins may increase the scrotal-testicular temperature, thereby diminishing the sperm quality. By cutting the veins, the scrotal temperature is restored to normal and fecundity may be improved.

Unfortunately, well-designed controlled studies have not shown any statistical increase in pregnancy rates following varicocelectomy. Furthermore, many fertile men have varicoceles. Today, this procedure is rarely, if ever, indicated. In most cases of male factor infertility, the best treatment involves intrauterine insemination (IUI) or, more often, proceeding directly with in vitro fertilization (IVF) and possibly intracytoplasmic sperm injection (ICSI).

31. What can cause my husband to have no sperm at all and can we still have children together?

Assuming that there was not a problem in collecting the specimen, the absence of sperm on a semen analysis—a condition known as **azoospermia**—requires thorough evaluation. Azoospermia can be divided into two major categories: obstructive and nonobstructive.

Obstructive azoospermia occurs when the duct carrying the sperm from the testicle to the urethra becomes blocked. This blockage may be the result of previous surgery on the scrotum or testicle, or even follow repair of an inguinal hernia. During hernia surgery, the vas deferens may be inadvertently damaged or even cut.

Azoospermia
The absence of sperm in a semen analysis.

Azoospermia can be divided into two major categories: obstructive and nonobstructive.

Scar tissue that blocks the vas deferens can form either postoperatively or as the result of an infection (most commonly gonorrhea, though other infectious diseases may also cause blockage of the sperm duct).

Some men are born without a vas deferens on either side. **Congenital bilateral absence of the vas deferens (CBAVD)** is associated with the gene for cystic fibrosis and is a rather unusual presentation of cystic fibrosis as it occurs in the absence of any chronic lung disease. For this reason, any man with azoospermia associated with congenital absence of the vas deferens should undergo genetic testing to determine whether he carries the gene that causes cystic fibrosis.

Congenital bilateral absence of the vas deferens (CBAVD)

Absence of the sperm-carrying duct in a man, resulting in azoospermia. This condition is frequently associated with cystic fibrosis.

Nonobstructive azoospermia results from dysfunctional sperm production as opposed to an anatomic issue and can represent a more problematic situation. The failure of sperm production in an otherwise normal testis may be the result of either a testicular issue or a pituitary or hypothalamus issue. If a hormonal evaluation reveals normal levels of prolactin and thyroid hormone, then testicular sperm production may have failed. If this finding is associated with an elevated FSH level, then the chance of finding any sperm production in the testis is quite unlikely. A testicular biopsy is often performed to assess whether any sperm are present within the testis. Even very low levels of sperm production may allow for attempts at IVF using ICSI. Genetic testing to rule out a chromosomal problem is often suggested in cases of very low or absent sperm production. We suggest that men undergoing a testicular biopsy arrange for cryopreservation (freezing) of viable sperm in order to avoid having to undergo a second biopsy procedure.

The use of IVF with ICSI can allow couples to successfully achieve pregnancy even in cases of obstructive or nonobstructive azoospermia. Sperm that is removed from the **epididymis** or the testicle may look excellent but is incapable of fertilizing an egg since it has not undergone the final changes that result in fully capacitated sperm. The introduction of ICSI in 1993 revolutionized the treatment of male factor infertility. To obtain sperm for use in IVF/ICSI, a needle aspiration of the testis or epididymis can be performed under local anesthesia in cases of obstructive azoospermia. If the male partner has nonobstructive azoospermia, a urologist usually performs a testicular biopsy in the hospital while the patient is under general anesthesia as sperm production may be severely impaired, necessitating the removal of more testicular tissue in order to have an adequate sample. In either case, the testicular tissue or the sperm aspirate can be frozen in liquid nitrogen and maintained relatively indefinitely. If a testicular biopsy reveals no mature sperm, then the only option is to use donor sperm or to pursue adoption.

Occasionally, the sperm retrieved through a testicular biopsy or needle aspiration is of exceedingly poor quality. In such cases, a repeat testicular biopsy on the day of **egg collection** for IVF or even use of a cryopreserved specimen from an anonymous sperm donor may be considered as a backup plan.

Rarely, men with diabetes or those taking certain antihypertensive medications may suffer from **retrograde ejaculation**. In this condition, there is no emission of fluid with male orgasm because all of the fluids travel backward into the bladder instead of out through the urethra. Retrograde ejaculation can easily be diagnosed by checking the post-ejaculation voided urine for sperm.

Specific Problems: Male Factors

Epididymis

Paired sac-like structures that are found atop each testicle and that serve as a repository for sperm prior to ejaculation.

Egg collection

A minimally invasive procedure usually performed transvaginally under minimal sedation in which eggs are removed from the ovaries.

Retrograde ejaculation

Backward movement of semen into the urinary bladder at the time of ejaculation.

Sperm present in the man's urine can be washed and used for either insemination or IVF. Pretreatment with bicarbonate the night before sperm collection may improve sperm quality by increasing the pH of the urine.

One final (and interesting) cause of azoospermia is anabolic steroid abuse. Some men with azoospermia may have used testosterone or other steroids as part of their strength and conditioning training. High doses of these steroids can suppress sperm production. Sperm production can be reinitiated in such patients by stopping the steroids and starting gonadotropin therapy (analogous to ovulation induction therapy in women). Although clomiphene citrate has been used to improve sperm quality in men, most studies reveal it to have little to no benefit.

32. Should I consider using a sperm donor to conceive?

Oligospermia

An abnormally low concentration of sperm in a semen analysis.

Couples who desire a child but in whom the male partner has a very low sperm count (**oligospermia**) or no sperm at all (azoospermia) often consider using third-party sperm donation and artificial insemination. Donor sperm can also be used by single women or lesbian couples. Many high-quality, reputable commercial sperm banks exist. They recruit and thoroughly test the donors and provide a listing of their available donors and their characteristics from which the couple can then choose. The donated sperm is obtained from the donor, tested, and quarantined for at least 6 months at the sperm bank. The donors are then retested to ensure that they are still free from any sexually transmitted diseases.

The specimen is released for use only after the test results confirm the donor is free from any infection.

The frozen sperm is then shipped to the physician's office, and artificial insemination is performed around the time of the woman's ovulation. Placement of the sperm inside the uterus (IUI) results in better pregnancy rates than placement of the sperm in the vagina or cervix. Frozen donor sperm can also be used for more advanced fertility procedures such as gonadotropin/IUI or IVF with or without ICSI. If a woman wishes to use sperm from a known donor with whom she does not have a physical relationship, then the sperm may need to be quarantined for at least 6 months and the donor retested for infectious diseases before the specimen can be used for fertility treatments. We strongly urge that all patients considering the use of a known sperm donor seek legal advice to ensure complete agreement of all parties involved.

Specific Problems: Male Factors

PART SIX

Specific Problems: Endometriosis

What is endometriosis and how
is it diagnosed?

Does surgery for endometriosis
improve pregnancy rates?

Are there medical treatments
for endometriosis?

More . . .

33. What is endometriosis and how is it diagnosed?

Endometriosis is a chronic disease characterized by the growth of endometrial-like tissue beyond the normal confines of the uterine cavity. Most commonly, it is located on the ovaries, but it can also be found on any of the organs inside the pelvic–abdominal cavities. Endometriosis is usually diagnosed at the time of laparoscopic gynecologic surgery although endometriosis cysts (endometriomas) may be presumptively diagnosed on ultrasound.

Although there are several theories about formation of endometriosis, it seems likely that retrograde menstruation (the passage of menstrual debris out of the ends of the fallopian tubes and into the pelvis) plays a major role. Some women may be unable to effectively remove this tissue, allowing lesions to form and grow with continued hormonal stimulation. Since the endometrium sheds through menstrual bleeding every month the endometrial tissue that comprises the endometriosis implants will also respond in kind. This phenomenon leads to inflammation of the pelvic reproductive organs, causing pelvic pain, painful periods (**dysmenorrhea**), and infertility. Pelvic adhesions or scar tissue may also develop. However, since endometriosis has been described in areas outside of the pelvis (eye, lung, brain, etc.), the retrograde menstruation theory cannot account for all cases of endometriosis.

Dysmenorrhea

Extremely painful periods.

Endometriosis may be suspected when patients complain of increasingly severe dysmenorrhea, pelvic pain, or infertility, but remember that it can be definitively diagnosed only via surgery. Most often, a diagnostic laparoscopy—a simple outpatient surgical procedure—is used to diagnose endometriosis. Other nonsurgical techniques such as ultrasonography, CT scan, or MRI can occasionally be helpful in their abilities to detect endometriosis.

34. Does surgery for endometriosis improve pregnancy rates?

Well-designed medical studies clearly show that destroying even small implants of endometriosis can improve fertility by as much as 50%. In a large Canadian study, the monthly pregnancy rate following surgical treatment of minimal endometriosis rose from 3% to 4.5%. Although this finding represented a 50% improvement in the patients' monthly chance of pregnancy, it does not compare very favorably with IVF pregnancy rates, which average above 30% for a single treatment cycle. Nevertheless, because treatment of endometriosis at the time of surgery does improve pregnancy rates, most surgeons will do their best to destroy endometriosis at the time of laparoscopy by using either laser or coagulation techniques. In addition to improving fertility, surgery may often eliminate or improve symptoms of dysmenorrhea and pelvic pain.

Ovarian cysts that contain endometriotic tissue may grow quite large. They are often called "chocolate cysts" because of the dark brown fluid found within them, although endometriosis cysts are more correctly referred to as endometriomas. If left untreated, these growths may destroy part or all of the normal ovarian tissue, including the eggs. Endometriomas must be surgically removed, usually via laparoscopy, as medical therapy is ineffective in the treatment of endometriomas. The ultimate choice of whether to perform a laparoscopy or laparotomy depends on the operative findings and the skill and experience of the surgeon.

35. Are there medical treatments for endometriosis?

Several medications are used to treat endometriosis. All of these medications suppress ovulation and cause a **hypoestrogenic** state. Understandably, suppressing ovulation also prevents pregnancy from occurring so medical therapy is not appropriate in patients actively seeking fertility. In patients who are not trying to conceive, medical treatment of endometriosis can be very beneficial and relieve symptoms of dysmenorrhea and pelvic pain.

One common medical treatment is to prescribe the combination oral contraceptive pill. Although each of these daily pills contains estrogen, the progestin (progesterone-like component) in the pill overrides the estrogen effect, resulting in suppression of endometriotic lesions. **Oral contraceptive pills** are effective in 30% to 60% of patients with endometriosis-related pain.

Many physicians prescribe **gonadotropin-releasing hormone (GnRH) analogs** (such as Lupron), which reduce estrogen levels to postmenopausal levels for their patients with endometriosis. These medications suppress estrogen production, prevent ovulation, and cause atrophy of the endometriosis in 70% to 90% patients. Unfortunately, GnRH analogs are expensive and must be given as injections either once a month or every 3 months. GnRH agonists can cause side effects including headaches, hot flashes, moodiness, insomnia, and vaginal dryness. To counteract these side effects experienced by many patients treated with GnRH agonists, physicians often prescribe oral contraceptive pills or supplemental progestin therapy (such as norethindrone) along with the GnRH analogs. This combined therapy may allow for improved treatment acceptance and alleviate many side effects associated with the use of the GnRH analogs as

Hypoestrogenic

A state of low estrogen.

Oral contraceptive pills

Daily medications, usually containing both synthetic estrogen and progesterone, that act as very effective contraceptives by suppressing follicle growth and ovulation.

Gonadotropin-releasing hormone (GnRH) analog

Medication that initially causes the pituitary gland to release its stores of follicle-stimulating hormone and luteinizing hormone, but that with continued use leads to markedly suppressed levels of these two hormones.

single therapy. Patients tolerate this combination very well and achieve maximal benefits in suppressing the disease and its symptoms.

As noted previously, medical therapy is not indicated for patients with endometriosis who are actively trying to conceive, since all of these treatments will suppress ovulation. Instead, for these patients, the goal should be to promptly establish pregnancy before the endometriosis causes any further damage to the reproductive organs. Generally, these women should seek treatment from a fertility expert to maximize their chances for successful pregnancy.

Medical therapy is not indicated for patients with endometriosis who are actively trying to conceive.

36. Do I need endometriosis surgery if I am already planning to pursue IVF?

The question of endometriosis surgery prior to IVF is a somewhat controversial area of reproductive medicine. Most reproductive endocrinologists do not recommend surgery prior to IVF unless the woman has advanced endometriosis, in particular, an ovarian endometrioma.

IVF is associated with excellent pregnancy rates (even without surgery) in women who have only mild to moderate endometriosis. When advanced endometriosis is present, such as an ovarian endometrioma, its surgical removal prior to IVF may enhance the chances for a successful IVF outcome and may decrease infectious complications related to egg collection. Thus, in such cases, most reproductive endocrinologists recommend the removal of advanced endometriosis prior to treatment using IVF.

However, severe endometriosis with endometriomas may lead to diminished ovarian responsiveness, and ovarian surgery may further compromise a patient's response to fertility drugs in such cases. So the decision to perform extensive surgery for endometriosis must be weighed against the potential impact of that surgery on the ovary.

Also, advanced endometriosis may increase the likelihood for an early pregnancy loss or spontaneous abortion. By first removing the endometriosis, the outcome of pregnancy may be improved. Ultimately, the decision whether or not to perform surgery rests between doctor and patient. In general, we believe that the removal of a small 1–2 cm endometrioma is unlikely to impact IVF success, but the removal of large endometriomas may be reasonable before attempting IVF. Some doctors advocate a threshold of 4 cm for endometrioma removal, but the data supporting this contention warrant further study.

Treatment Options: Intrauterine Insemination (IUI)

How do I know if IUI is an option for me and should I use fertility drugs in conjunction with an IUI?

What are typical pregnancy rates for IUI?

What complications can occur after IUI?

More . . .

37. What is the difference (if any) between intrauterine insemination and artificial insemination?

Artificial insemination (AI) is a historical term that encompasses any technique involving the introduction of sperm into the female reproductive tract without sexual intercourse. Semen can be placed into the vagina (intravaginal insemination) or into the cervix (**intracervical insemination**) without any special preparation of the specimen. However, if unprepared semen is placed directly into the uterus (intrauterine insemination (IUI)), then severe spasmodic uterine cramping can occur. Thus, when performing an IUI, the sperm must first be washed and prepared prior to placement inside the uterus. Washing the sperm removes the prostaglandins that cause the violent uterine contractions. Washing also eliminates substances that might lower the sperm quality and activates the sperm, thereby leading to improved sperm motility. Generally, the IUI specimen is prepared in the doctor's office just prior to insemination.

The actual IUI is a painless, simple, in-office procedure that is often performed by a nurse. It usually takes just a minute to perform. Physicians typically ask patients to come in with a full bladder so that the angle between the uterus and cervix is altered, which allows for easy passage of the catheter into the uterine cavity.

Today, it is rare for patients to undergo other forms of insemination besides IUI because the pregnancy rates with IUI are better than those obtained by intravaginal insemination or intracervical insemination.

Intracervical insemination

A fertility treatment in which sperm are placed within the cervix.

38. How do I know if IUI is an option for me and should I use fertility drugs in conjunction with an IUI?

IUI is a good option for many infertile couples. It can be performed in conjunction with a woman's natural cycle or can be combined with the use of fertility drugs. IUI can also be effectively used in couples who have sexual dysfunction or infrequent coitus for either medical or nonmedical reasons. For example, some couples may have busy work schedules such that one or the other partner is frequently out of town around the time of ovulation. If the male partner's sperm is obtained and cryopreserved (frozen) in advance of ovulation, the physician (or nurse) can perform an IUI and, ideally, facilitate pregnancy without the woman missing a menstrual cycle.

The best candidates for IUI are those couples without tubal disease or severe male factor infertility. Women with severe endometriosis or a history of pelvic adhesions are not good candidates for IUI. Although couples with male factor infertility can attempt IUI, the success rates are fairly low in such cases, and prompt consideration should be given to IVF (and ICSI) if pregnancy fails to occur after three or four attempts.

IUI, in combination with fertility medications, may provide a reasonable treatment option for some patients. There appears to be a synergistic benefit to the combination of fertility medications (either Clomid or injectable gonadotropins) with IUI compared to either treatment by itself. For this reason, most infertility experts recommend IUI to their patients when treating them with fertility drugs even if the semen analysis is normal.

Treatment Options: Intrauterine Insemination (IUI)

In women who fail to ovulate regularly, the goal of drug therapy is to induce the growth and release of a single mature egg. This treatment is known as ovulation induction. In contrast, the treatment goal for women with regular menstrual cycles is to induce the growth of multiple follicles with the subsequent release of multiple eggs. Hence the term **superovulation** (also called **controlled ovarian hyperstimulation**) is used to describe this treatment. During a cycle of superovulation and IUI, the goal is to develop 3 to 5 mature follicles, whereas the goal in an IVF cycle is to produce more.

Clomid is usually the fertility drug of first choice for both ovulation induction and superovulation with IUI. Women who fail to respond to Clomid or who fail to conceive may be candidates for treatment with injectable fertility medications (gonadotropins) combined with IUI. In some cases, it is best to skip the treatment with Clomid and instead proceed directly with gonadotropin therapy; this decision depends on the severity of the couple's infertility situation.

In women who have normal menstrual cycles, it would appear on the surface that IUI alone without fertility drugs would be as successful as IUI with fertility drugs. Unfortunately, this simply is not the case. Instead, the combination of IUI and fertility drugs to induce superovulation yields a synergistic benefit over either treatment alone. However, superovulation (either with or without IUI) can lead to multiple pregnancy. Historically, nearly all of the multiples (such as sextuplets and more) have been the result of superovulation. Unfortunately, there is really no way to control the outcome of this game of reproductive Russian Roulette. Patients must understand that if there are more than two follicles present, then the possibility of a high order multiple

Superovulation

The development of multiple ovarian follicles in response to fertility medication.

Controlled ovarian hyperstimulation

Stimulation of the ovaries with fertility medications to help them grow and release multiple eggs.

The combination of IUI and fertility drugs to induce superovulation yields a synergistic benefit over either treatment alone.

pregnancy is a reality. In such cases, a frank discussion with the patient needs to be held to review the risk and alternatives to avoid a poor outcome.

Rebecca comments:

I began actively seeking treatment for my infertility issues at the age of 40. My RE was very open with me and explained the limitations of IUI (in combination with injectable gonadotropins) for a woman my age. However, my husband and I opted to go through two IUI/injects cycles before we moved on to IVF. Despite the fact that IUI didn't work for us, our IUI experience was helpful for the RE, as well as for my husband and me. The RE could see how I responded to the medications and he used these experiences to develop our IVF protocol. For my husband and me, the IUI provided us with a less invasive and costly way (as compared to IVF) to be proactive in addressing our infertility issues. It was a good way to 'ease' into the process of medical intervention. We experienced the shots, being at monitoring appointments, having bloods drawn, getting to know the fertility center staff/routine, and the process of getting my husband's 'contribution.' And when the cycles failed, we experienced the sting and frustration of treatment failure. I know that for us, going through the IUIs prepared us for our subsequent IVFs.

39. What are typical pregnancy rates for IUI?

The pregnancy rates for IUI vary widely, depending mostly on the female partner's age and the presence or absence of any other infertility factors. In patients younger than 35 years old, an estimated one-third to one-half of patients will achieve pregnancy within 1 to 4 treatments. In patients with unexplained infertility, most studies demonstrate a per-cycle pregnancy rate of

6% for the Clomid/IUI combination and 9% to 12% for the gonadotropin/IUI combination, compared with a spontaneous pregnancy rate of less than 5% per month (see **Table 3**). Many fertility doctors will try 1 to 4 cycles of Clomid/IUI and then 1 to 4 cycles of gonadotropin/IUI. If pregnancy has not occurred after the fourth treatment, most experts would abandon these treatments and proceed with more aggressive therapy such as in vitro fertilization. The optimal number of IUI treatment cycles should be individually determined by the patient and her infertility specialist.

Some patients develop a seeming resistance to fertility medications, demonstrating reduced responses with repeated stimulations. This problem is especially prevalent in women who are more than 37 years old. Thus, in our opinion, IVF should be considered as a first-line treatment in these patients as opposed to multiple gonadotropin/IUI cycles.

Table 3   Unexplained Infertility Success Rates Per Cycle with Various Treatment Options

Method	Pregnancy Rate (%)
Intercourse	4
IUI	4
CC	5.6
CC + IUI	8
FSH	7.7
FSH + IUI	17
In vitro fertilization	21

CC, clomiphene citrate; FSH, follicle-stimulating hormone; IUI, intrauterine insemination.
Source: Adapted from Guzick DS, et al. Efficacy of treatment for unexplained infertility. *Fertil Steril* 70:207, 1998.

40. How many office visits are required during a typical cycle using fertility drugs and IUI?

For treatments using Clomid and IUI, only a couple of office visits per month are required. Clomid is usually prescribed at doses of 50–100 mg daily taken on cycle days 5–9. We typically have patients begin monitoring on cycle day 12. At a typical office visit for monitoring, the patient has her blood drawn for hormone analysis, and a pelvic ultrasound is performed to measure the size of the follicles and the thickness of the endometrial lining. The doctor uses this information to determine the optimal timing of the HCG trigger shot and the subsequent IUI. Most patients receive the HCG trigger injection once the follicle size is >20–22 mm mean diameter. This trigger shot will induce ovulation around 36–40 hours later so the IUI is scheduled accordingly or the couple is informed of the best timing for intercourse. Occasionally a patient will demonstrate an LH surge on her own and the timing of the IUI or coitus should take this into account.

For treatment using gonadotropins and IUI, closer monitoring is necessary, perhaps requiring 4 to 6 office visits per treatment cycle. Patients in our practice undergo a baseline sonogram on cycle days 2 or 3 to rule out any persistent ovarian cysts from the preceding treatment cycle. If the sonogram is normal, then patients begin the daily injections and usually return to the office after 3–4 days of medication to assess the response to the drugs. Adjustments in the dose of the medications may allow for the optimal treatment response and most patients require 10–12 days of shots before the follicles reach the ideal size. Once again, the HCG trigger shot is used to induce ovulation at the appropriate time and the IUI is scheduled accordingly. The actual IUI takes only minutes to perform and is usually painless. We routinely ask our patients to lie on their backs for about 10 to 15 minutes following the IUI procedure. The woman may then return to her normal activities. In couples pursuing timed intercourse, a pregnancy test is performed, usually 14 days following an IUI or 16 days following HCG.

41. I read on the Internet that two inseminations are better than one. Is this true?

In general, one well-timed IUI is as good as two, and no advantage is obtained by performing a second IUI (providing ovulation was well monitored using blood hormone determinations and follicle ultrasound measurements). However, in patients who are undergoing IUI with less intense monitoring of ovulation, such as urine LH testing, or for those women who chose not to monitor their ovulation at all, two inseminations may be a better option.

Using basal body temperatures as the basis for an IUI's timing is not recommended, because this method cannot prospectively pinpoint the optimal timing of ovulation for an IUI treatment. The rise in basal body temperature occurs after ovulation, so identifying this temperature increase would not help in scheduling an IUI procedure.

42. Can we have sex during a treatment cycle?

In general, the answer is yes. Many experts, however, recommend no coitus for 2 to 3 days prior to an anticipated IUI to "build up" the male partner's sperm count and volume. Also, some men may experience difficulty producing a specimen if they have recently had coitus. For men who have a low sperm count or motility, it is recommended that they abstain from sexual relations for 3 to 5 days prior to a planned IUI. In patients who are at risk for hyperstimulation syndrome, it may be wise to refrain from sex until the ovarian response has been assessed. In patients with an excessive response to fertility drugs the cycle may be abandoned and yet ovulation could still occur. Since the sperm can survive up to 5–7 days after intercourse, a pregnancy could occur even in the setting of a cancelled IUI or IVF cycle.

Men who have a low sperm count or motility, it is recommended that they abstain from sexual relations for 3 to 5 days prior to a planned IUI.

43. My doctor wants to use Lupron or Antagon during my IUI cycle. What are these drugs, and why do I need them? I thought they were only for IVF.

Lupron and Antagon are injectable medications that are used to prevent premature release of LH hormone during a stimulation cycle for IUI or IVF. These two medications work through different mechanisms to prevent the LH surge. Lupron usually requires at least 7 days to effectively prevent an LH surge, whereas Antagon works within hours. This difference explains why the drug protocols that employ these two medications are so different. Premature ovulation during an IUI cycle can be dealt with by simply adjusting the timing of the IUI, so these medications are primarily used in patients undergoing IVF rather than IUI. For most patients undergoing treatment with IUI these medications are not needed unless a patient repeatedly experiences a premature LH surge during the treatment cycle. In such cases, these medications can allow for a more optimal stimulation and larger follicle sizes.

44. What complications can occur after IUI?

Complications related to the actual IUI procedure are very rare. IUI is a simple, in-office, nonsurgical procedure, usually performed by nurses. Occasionally, patients may experience mild to moderate uterine cramps as the catheter is passed through the cervix into their uterus. These cramps usually last 10 to 15 minutes. Infection rarely occurs (its incidence is less than 1%). Many infertility specialists routinely obtain cervical cultures prior to initiating an IUI cycle, and the culture media used to prepare the IUI specimen commonly contains antibiotics. Occasionally, patients may note some light spotting after placement of the IUI catheter, but this is not an indication of a complication or a problem. Multiple pregnancy can occur in any situation when two or more mature follicles are present at the time of HCG. Your physician should discuss with you the risk of multiple pregnancy in cycles using fertility medication to induce the growth of multiple follicles. Similarly, patients with an excessive response to fertility medication can also be at risk for ovarian hyperstimulation syndrome (OHSS). However, both multiple gestation and OHSS can result from the stimulation of the ovary with hormones regardless of whether an IUI is performed or not.

Multiple pregnancy can occur in any situation when two or more mature follicles are present at the time of HCG.

45. How would I know when to pursue more advanced fertility treatments?

The decision to seek out more advanced fertility treatments is a complex question, and multiple factors must be considered when making it. For most couples undergoing treatment with IUI (either alone or with fertility drugs), the best chances for success usually occur within the first four treatment cycles. After that, the likelihood for pregnancy decreases. In many of our patients, we recommend only one or two IUI treatments. If these efforts are unsuccessful, we suggest that the couple proceed with other, more aggressive treatments, including both Natural Cycle IVF and traditional IVF using injectable fertility medications.

For some patients, IUI should rarely be utilized. For example, those couples with severe tubal disease, severe endometriosis, pelvic adhesions, or severe male factor infertility may do best by directly proceeding with IVF as their first treatment option. If an age factor is present or if the couple has prolonged infertility (infertility lasting more than 5 years), we often recommend IVF first, as well. Remember that IVF is the only treatment for which even a failed treatment cycle provides some insight into a couple's fertility potential. IVF does allow us to make some assessment of egg quality, fertilization and embryo development. A failed IUI cycle yields no such information as we only know that the cycle failed but learn nothing about fertilization, embryo growth or embryo quality.

PART EIGHT

Treatment Options: In Vitro Fertilization (IVF)

What is IVF, and how is it performed?

How successful is IVF?

Are there age or other restrictions on who should do IVF?

More . . .

46. *What is IVF, and how is it performed?*

In vitro fertilization (IVF) was first successfully performed in Oldham, England, in 1978, resulting in the birth of Louise Brown, who was conceived using Natural Cycle IVF (NC-IVF). Since then, more than 4 million children have been born using IVF. The introduction of this technique completely changed—and greatly improved—our ability to treat even the most difficult cases of infertility, many of which were previously untreatable. Although it is clearly not a "cure-all" for infertility, IVF has revolutionized our approach to, and understanding of, the disease called infertility.

IVF literally means "the fertilization of eggs with sperm in glass," which translates to fertilization outside of the body in the laboratory. There are two types of IVF: (1) stimulated cycle IVF, and (2) Natural Cycle IVF (NC-IVF). We will focus on stimulated cycle IVF in this question but for more information on NC-IVF, please refer to Question 59). An IVF cycle consists of several discrete phases, as detailed in the sections that follow.

Phase 1: Ovarian Stimulation

A woman's ovaries contain thousands of fluid-filled sacs called follicles. Inside each follicle is an egg (or ovum). In a normal reproductive cycle, only a single follicle (and egg) reaches maturity. Louise Brown (the world's first IVF baby) was produced in a natural cycle from a single follicle. Although a few clinics in the United States (including our own) remain enthusiastic about NC-IVF, most IVF in the United States is performed in a stimulated cycle using injectable fertility medications. The introduction of these medications (called gonadotropins) enabled physicians to increase the efficiency of IVF through the production of multiple mature follicles. Two forms of these medications are used: (1) drugs containing equal parts of the pituitary hormones follicle-stimulating hormone (FSH) and luteinizing hormone (LH) (Menopur), or (2) drugs containing only FSH (Bravelle, Gonal-F, Follistim) or LH (Luveris). Both kinds of medications induce the growth of multiple ovarian follicles, so it is important to monitor the woman's response to them carefully with ultrasound and blood hormone testing.

Estrogen is produced within each of the developing follicles and induces the growth of the lining of the uterus (endometrium). Unfortunately, the rise in estrogen can also induce the pituitary gland to prematurely trigger ovulation, resulting in the cancellation of an IVF cycle. Two other classes of drugs are used to reduce the chance of this problem occurring during an IVF stimulation: (1) GnRH agonists (such as Lupron and Synarel), and (2) GnRH antagonists (such as Centrotide and Antagon). Lupron (or Synarel) is usually started 1 week prior to the woman's anticipated next menstrual cycle. Given that a patient may have spontaneously conceived during this cycle, all women beginning Lupron are recommended to use a barrier form of contraception.

Approximately 1 week after starting Lupron, a woman should experience a normal menstrual period. An ultrasound exam is performed at the start of this menstrual cycle to examine the ovaries and measure any existing cysts. In some cases, empty follicles from a previous cycle will persist and may influence the response to FSH. If the baseline ultrasound and blood tests are normal, then the patient receives instructions that afternoon as to when and what dose of medication she should take and when she should report back to the office for repeat ultrasound and blood tests.

Patients remain on Lupron to prevent the premature release of the eggs until the end of the stimulation phase. During a typical treatment cycle, they take daily injections for 9 to 12 days before the follicles reach maturity based on ultrasound results and blood hormone levels. Once the follicles reach a 20- to 24-mm diameter, the woman receives an injection of human chorionic gonadotropin (HCG; Pregnyl, Profasi, Novaryl) at a precise time. This hormone serves as a trigger to incite the final maturation and release of the egg (ovulation). Ovulation typically occurs about 40 hours after this shot, so the egg collection procedure is scheduled for 34–36 hours after the HCG injection. Failure to take the HCG will result in an egg collection with apparently empty follicles as the eggs will not be ready for aspiration or eggs that are retrieved will be immature. Clearly, taking the HCG is absolutely critical which is why we check a blood test for HCG the morning after the shot to ensure that it was given correctly.

Cycles using GnRH antagonists are somewhat different. GnRH antagonists are started several days following the start of ovarian stimulation with gonadotropins. Most clinics add the GnRH antagonist once the largest follicle reaches a diameter of 14 mm. This medication effectively prevents the release of LH from the pituitary within hours of administration. Although many clinics have used GnRH antagonists successfully as part of their IVF stimulation protocols, some studies have demonstrated a trend toward decreased implantation rates in IVF cycles using this class of medications. Some physicians use GnRH agonists (Lupron) instead of HCG to induce follicular maturation. This approach only works in patients who have not already been taking Lupron as part of their stimulation protocol.

Phase 2: Oocyte Retrieval

Many physicians perform IVF as an office-based procedure, whereas others utilize a free-standing surgery center. Some programs are located within a hospital. There are advantages and disadvantages to each of these. We prefer to perform egg collections at our office in a special procedure room, as the location and staff are familiar to the patients undergoing the IVF process. We also find that the location of the IVF lab within the office encourages continuous communication between patient, physician, and embryology staff. However, clearly many successful programs utilize a surgery center or a hospital. The use of a hospital setting may allow patients with significant medical conditions (cardiac disease, severe pulmonary disease) to undergo IVF, whereas such patients would be considered an anesthesia risk in the office setting.

Although many patients are nervous about the oocyte retrieval, in fact the vast majority of women find it to be less uncomfortable than some of the screening tests leading up to IVF. The egg collection is performed under intravenous sedation using a vaginal ultrasound probe with a special needle guide adapter. Most patients have no recollection of the actual egg retrieval and sleep through the entire procedure. The needle passes through the side of the vagina into the ovary, and the follicles are easily aspirated. The fluid containing the eggs is then inspected by the **embryologist** using a microscope. Both the eggs and the sperm are then placed together in small plastic dishes containing media and incubated for the next 3 to 5 days. If there is a significant male factor, then ICSI (see Question 53) is performed several hours after the egg collection.

Embryologist

A scientist involved in the fertilization and culture of human eggs and embryos.

Phase 3: Embryo Culture

On the day following the egg collection, patients learn how many eggs were fertilized. Remember that although your RE measures all of the follicles during stimulation, mature eggs are usually found only in follicles with a diameter of more than 17 mm. In general, about 70% of the mature eggs will fertilize. Unfortunately, some attrition occurs at each point in an IVF cycle so the total number of healthy embryos is often much less than the original number of follicles or eggs.

Three days after the egg collection procedure, the embryos selected for embryo transfer will be identified. Allowing the embryos to grow for an additional 2–3 days in the laboratory may allow for enhanced embryo selection as some excellent appearing day 3 embryos will fail to continue to grow. Thus, implantation rates are usually higher for day 5–6 transfers because of this improved ability to select the best embryos. Additionally, there is some evidence that suggests waiting until day 5–6 may provide for improved synchronization of embryo and endometrium given that, in nature, the embryo usually doesn't arrive in the uterus until day 5–6 after ovulation. On the day of embryo transfer, your RE should review the quantity and quality of the embryos with the embryologist and then discuss with you his or her recommendations regarding the number of embryos to transfer.

Embryos that are not selected for transfer may still be of excellent quality, so they may be candidates for cryopreservation (freezing) with liquid nitrogen. These frozen embryos can then be replaced into the uterus during a future cycle, eliminating the need for the woman to undergo the entire IVF process of ovarian stimulation and egg collection. There is little benefit to freezing poor-quality embryos, however, because they are unlikely to result in a pregnancy and may not even survive the thawing process.

Phase 4: Embryo Transfer

Embryo transfer is one of the most critical aspects of an IVF cycle. During this phase, the embryos are transferred into the uterus by a procedure similar to an IUI. At our office, we perform our embryo transfers under abdominal ultrasound guidance to ensure the accurate placement of the embryos into the uterus. On the day of embryo transfer, patients are asked to drink 48 ounces of water and keep a full bladder to enable us to visualize the transfer of the embryos. No anesthesia is usually required for an embryo transfer and this step usually takes only 1–2 minutes to complete.

Phase 5: Post-Transfer and Pregnancy

During the 2 weeks after the embryo transfer, patients take supplemental progesterone (shots and/or suppositories). If a patient's estrogen level drops significantly during the 2 weeks following embryo transfer, her physician may add supplemental estrogen as well.

Two weeks after the transfer, the woman typically undergoes a blood pregnancy test. Once a pregnancy test is positive, the physician may repeat the test every 2 days until the beta HCG level is high enough to visualize the pregnancy sac on transvaginal ultrasound (the beta HCG level should be more than 2000 IU around 3 to 4 weeks following embryo transfer). A follow-up ultrasound is then performed to confirm fetal cardiac activity. At this point, patients are usually referred back to their obstetrician/gynecologist for prenatal care.

Two weeks after the transfer, the woman typically undergoes a blood pregnancy test.

Carol comments:

Before undergoing IVF, I remember thinking that Phases 1 through 4 would be the hardest part. I was very intimidated by all the drugs and the shots and the egg collection. In reality, it was Phase 5 that was the toughest. I had done everything I could do—mixed the drugs, given the shots, drank the water. Now all that was left was to wait and see if it worked.

One piece of helpful advice I was given was to plan something out of the ordinary during those 2 weeks. Whether it's a vacation with your husband or visiting a relative, introducing anything that is not part of your normal routine is helpful in keeping your mind off of whether or not you're pregnant.

47. How do I know if I need IVF?

Not all patients need IVF or are good candidates for IVF. Thus, the answer to this question can be determined only after you undergo a comprehensive infertility evaluation by your reproductive endocrinologist. Nevertheless, some situations clearly require the use of IVF. For example, women with absent or severely damaged fallopian tubes should be treated immediately with IVF. Likewise, IVF should be performed first if the male partner has very poor sperm quality. For other patients, the use of IVF may be less clear-cut, especially given that many different treatment options exist. In such cases, the doctor should discuss with the couple the pros and cons of each option, and then all parties should jointly decide on a treatment plan.

Kristin comments:

After I lost my right fallopian tube to an ectopic pregnancy, we discussed the various ART options with our RE.

Due to my PCOS diagnosis as well as having only one tube, my chance of conceiving during an IUI cycle was around 10% at best, whereas my chance of conceiving via IVF was significantly higher than a typical 30-year-old fertile woman's chance. We were eager to start our family and decided to go with the more aggressive treatment because it had a higher success rate. It helped that our insurance covered the procedure. I think it is important to know the success rates for the treatment options your RE suggests. When given the choice between a 10% chance of conceiving through IUI and a more than 50% chance of conceiving through IVF, the choice seemed clear.

48. How successful is IVF?

Overall, the success rates for IVF have improved markedly since 1978 (when Louise Brown was conceived), but success rates vary widely depending on the couple's infertility factors and the clinic performing the IVF procedure (see **Table 4**). Success rates for U.S. IVF clinics are published on the CDC's website (www.cdc.gov/ART/ index.htm). The standardization of clinic success rates evolved from 1994 passage of the Fertility Clinic Success Rate and Certification Act (the so-called **Wyden law**), which seeks to protect U.S. consumers from inflated IVF success rates. Importantly, many subtleties influence clinic-specific IVF pregnancy rates, including

Success rates for U.S. IVF clinics are published on the CDC's website (www.cdc.gov/ART/ index.htm).

Wyden law

Legislation passed by the U.S. Congress and sponsored by Congressman Ron Wyden that regulates the advertising and reporting of IVF success rates by fertility clinics.

Table 4   Factors Influencing IVF Success Rates

1. Patient's age
2. Type of infertility diagnosis
3. Duration of infertility (Best prognosis if <5yrs)
4. Experience/expertise of the clinic
5. Number of embryos transferred
6. Type of IVF performed: Stimulated vs. Natural Cycle IVF

patient selection bias (that is, some clinics tend to treat tougher cases, so their success rates might be lower than those of clinics that take only routine cases). The paucity of clinics that offer Natural Cycle IVF (NC-IVF) is likely related to this reporting requirement. NC-IVF can be an effective fertility treatment but the pregnancy rate will be less than for stimulated cycle IVF and the number of cancelled cycles will also be higher as patients may ovulate before egg collection, or fail to fertilize or fail to have a viable embryo to transfer.

Unfortunately, at the present time all IVF cycles are reported the same way with the CDC failing to segregate results from NC-IVF from stimulated cycle IVF. Needless to say, this reporting method does not encourage clinics to offer NC-IVF as the apparent IVF success rate will be reduced by the inclusion of NC-IVF in the calculations.

For women younger than 34 years of age, most will achieve pregnancy within 1 to 3 treatment cycles; indeed, many succeed in their first attempt. For women older than 35 years, the success rates tend to decrease simply because the aging process affects the quality of these women's eggs. For a detailed discussion of IVF success rates, couples should visit the website for the clinic where they are considering treatment. They should also discuss their specific likelihood of success with their reproductive endocrinologist. IVF pregnancy rates do vary by clinic, so patients should carefully scrutinize their chances for success at the particular clinic rendering treatment.

Carol comments:

This was one part of the process that I found to be a bit more predictable. In both my pregnancies, it took two IVF attempts to achieve a viable pregnancy. As tough as it was after each failed attempt, I tried to take something positive away. For example, after my very first IVF attempt resulted in a chemical pregnancy, I focused on the fact that I now knew an embryo could implant in the lining of my uterus. When I was trying to get pregnant the second time, I did a FET [frozen embryo transfer] with frozen embryos from the previous cycle. Again, it resulted in a chemical pregnancy. Based on that experience, we decided that we would not pursue another FET. I am convinced that maintaining a positive attitude during the process makes a big difference.

49. Are the children born after IVF normal?

The question of the health of children born after advanced fertility treatments is one that has great importance both to patients and fertility physicians alike. In general, the data regarding the outcomes for children born after IVF, either with or without the use of ICSI, have been extremely reassuring.

The problem with these studies is the identification of an appropriate control group with which to compare the rate of problems found in the children conceived with advanced fertility techniques. Overall, most studies suggest a background risk of birth defects in naturally conceived children of approximately 4% to 5%. However, these couples tend to be younger than the couples undergoing IVF and, by definition, do not suffer from infertility. Although the vast majority of studies suggest no increased risk of anomalies in children conceived after IVF, few of these studies have looked at the rate of congenital anomalies in children conceived naturally but born to parents who suffered infertility that spontaneously

The vast majority of studies suggest no increased risk of anomalies in children conceived after IVF.

resolved without treatment. This group of patients clearly represents a more appropriate control group with which to compare patients who seek out advanced fertility treatments. The few studies that have looked at this question have noted that although patients who suffered from infertility have a higher rate of anomalies and pregnancy related complications, the means by which these couples eventually conceived (spontaneously or with IVF) did not influence the rate of these problems. Therefore, it may not be the IVF process per se that is the issue here but rather the underlying infertility that matters.

Recently, in Australia, a systematic review was conducted of all studies that had previously examined the possible increased risk to children conceived after treatment with IVF and/or ICSI (Hansen, M. et al., Human Reproduction. 20 (2):328–338, 2005). However, many of these studies compare the rate of congenital abnormalities in children conceived spontaneously with the rate in children who were born to older couples undergoing IVF and/or ICSI. In many studies, the rate of congenital anomalies in the control group has been around 4%, whereas the rate of congenital anomalies in the group of couples undergoing IVF and ICSI has been 6% or greater. The difference between 4% and 6% is statistically significant and suggests that there may be an increased risk to children conceived through the use of advanced reproductive techniques. However, the question still remains as to whether this is a problem related to IVF itself or to the underlying infertility that leads to the use of IVF. In any case, most patients accept an increased absolute risk of 2% as being reasonable, especially given that their options for spontaneous conception may be significantly limited.

The greatest risk to the children conceived after fertility treatment is that of prematurity related to multiple pregnancy. Several strategies are used to reduce the rate of multiple gestations (see Question 50). The risks of prematurity associated with twins are significant and should not be discounted quickly, especially given that 50% of twins deliver a month or more before their due date.

In addition, the question has been raised as to whether even IVF singleton pregnancies are at higher risk for low birth weight and prematurity. If true, the cause of this increased risk may be difficult to determine. Patients undergoing IVF suffer from infertility, so any increased rate of adverse pregnancy outcome might not be so much a result of the IVF process as it is related to the couple's underlying problem of infertility. Several studies have suggested that women who conceive spontaneously, but who have a preceding history of infertility, have a significantly increased rate of prematurity and pregnancy-related complications such as placenta previa, abruption, and low-birth-weight infants.

Another way to look at the question of whether any risk is related to the process of IVF itself versus the patient population undergoing IVF is to examine the pregnancy outcomes in women who undergo IVF but use a **gestational carrier** (carriers usually have an excellent reproductive history). A study of these pregnancies found there was no increased risk of prematurity or low birth weight in the children conceived and carried in this way. This reassuring outcome would suggest that the problem lies not so much with the IVF process but, unfortunately, with the patients who require IVF to conceive.

The greatest risk to the children conceived after fertility treatment is that of prematurity related to multiple pregnancy.

Treatment Options: In Vitro Fertilization (IVF)

Gestational carrier

A woman who undergoes an embryo transfer consisting of an embryo produced by another couple (or from donor gametes) with the intention to give the resulting baby back to the genetic parents.

The impact of new and emerging technologies on the rate of congenital anomalies in children born after fertility treatment remains a subject of ongoing debate. The potential risks inherent in micromanipulation of the embryo prior to embryo transfer—like that required for preimplantation genetic diagnosis (PGD)—remain unknown. Although more than 4 million IVF babies have been delivered worldwide to date, only a relatively small number of children have been delivered after the use of PGD or following unusual situations such as "rescue ICSI" performed on the day following egg collection because of unanticipated failed fertilization. When considering such novel treatments, the physician needs to inform the patient/couple of any known or suspected risks. Currently, several studies are under way in this country and throughout the world to continue to monitor the health of those children delivered following advanced fertility treatments.

Carol comments:

Although this question is focused on the "physical normalcy" of IVF babies, I would like to comment on the "perceived normalcy" of IVF babies. I do understand that a large percentage of people will never have to deal with this challenge, and that ignorance is bliss, but I am still surprised by how commonplace the misperceptions related to ART are.

I'll never forget a comment that a woman made to me during my first pregnancy. I was flying back from a visit with my extended family during which we had announced the long-awaited news that I was pregnant. My husband and I struck up a conversation with the woman sitting next to us. As what now seems inevitable, the subject of IVF came up. I confirmed that my pregnancy was, indeed, a result of IVF. Without missing a beat, the woman looked at me and said, "I've never seen one of those babies." I was astounded.

Luckily, my husband was there to help me regain my composure and politely explain to the woman that, in fact, IVF babies are not from Mars. Long story short, it's hard to anticipate what people might say to you, so be prepared.

50. How do I decide how many embryos to transfer?

Determining the number of embryos to transfer in an IVF cycle is a crucial decision that requires careful discussion between the patient/couple and the physician. The goal of every treatment cycle should be the delivery of a full-term, healthy, singleton baby. Although transferring more than one embryo will increase the pregnancy rate, at some point transferring additional embryos merely serves to increase the multiple pregnancy rate without altering the overall pregnancy rate. Several European countries have eliminated all discussion of how many embryos to transfer by mandating that all patients undergo only single-embryo transfers. Whereas elective (or mandatory) single-embryo transfer has been promoted heavily throughout Europe, it has not yet received widespread acceptance in the United States, although this attitude may be changing slowly.

The goal of every treatment cycle should be the delivery of a full-term, healthy, singleton baby.

One of the major disadvantages of single-embryo transfer is that it leads to a decreased IVF pregnancy rate from the fresh cycle. Proponents of single-embryo transfer claim that the potential reduction in the overall pregnancy rate is well worth the marked reduction in the twin pregnancy rate. Twin pregnancies can be problematic because they are associated with higher rates of preterm labor and preterm delivery. Some couples, however, may desire twins or at least regard them as a neutral outcome. This view is especially prevalent among patients who are paying for the treatment themselves (rather than it being covered by insurance) and regard twins as a "two for the price of one" outcome. As noted in Question 49, the greatest risk to the health of children following IVF is the complications related to prematurity associated with multiple births. Despite the risks associated with multiple pregnancy, couples still tell us every day that they would "love to have twins."

In the United States, there is no question that the trend is to transfer a single embryo in most patients. We fully embrace this concept. In fact, with the recent advances in embryo cryopreservation, such as vitrification (see Question 72) frozen-thawed embryos seem to be as likely to implant and produce healthy pregnancies as embryos transferred in a fresh cycle. Thus, in the patients classified as "Most favorable prognosis" we see no need to transfer more than a single embryo and risk a multiple pregnancy when we can safely perform a frozen-thawed embryo using high-quality vitrified embryos. However, convincing patients has proved more difficult. One of the advantages of Natural Cycle IVF is that there is rarely the option to transfer more than a single embryo since nearly all patients produce only a single mature egg in a typical reproductive cycle. Some patients who had planned to undergo single embryo transfer will change their minds at the last minute and elect to transfer two embryos, greatly increasing the risk of a twin pregnancy. With Natural Cycle IVF the temptation to transfer two embryos has been eliminated entirely.

The ASRM has published guidelines for making the decision of how many embryos to transfer (see **Table 5**). Patients who fall into the excellent prognosis category should transfer only one or two embryos, whereas those with an exceedingly poor prognosis—because of the woman's age or multiple failed IVFs, for example—may undergo embryo transfer of five or more embryos.

Table 5   Recommended Limits on the Numbers of Embryos to Transfer

	Age			
Prognosis	< 35 yrs	35–37 yrs	38–40 yrs	41–42 yrs
Cleavage-stage embryos[a]				
Favorable[b] All others	1–2 2	2 3	3 4	5 5
Blastocysts[a]				
Favorable[b] All others	1 2	2 2	2 3	3 3

[a] Justification for transferring one additional embryo more than the recommended limit should be clearly documented in the patient's medical record.

[b] Favorable = first cycle of IVF, good embryo quality, excess embryos available for cryopreservation, or previous successful IVF cycle.

Source: Adapted from Guidelines on the number of embryos transferred. The Practice Committee of the Society for Assisted Reproductive Technology and the American Society for Reproductive Medicine. *Fertil Steril* 2009:92:1518-19. Copyright 2009 American Society for Reproductive Medicine.

The most problematic decisions concern those patients who fall between these two extremes. Couples who are paying out of pocket for IVF will often pressure their RE to be more aggressive in terms of the number of embryos transferred. Of course, the expense involved in caring for premature infants is many times greater than the cost of all of the fertility procedures used to initiate those pregnancies. The financial costs are merely one part of the picture, as caring for patients with preterm labor or premature infants is also associated with a variety of emotional, psychological, and physical costs.

If multiple pregnancies occur, a multifetal selective reduction procedure can be considered. This procedure is performed at approximately 10 weeks of pregnancy and involves injecting a salt solution into one or more of the gestational sacs. The overall pregnancy loss rate following this procedure is usually less than 5%. In patients who wish to avoid a triplet gestation (but who will not consider selective reduction), it is best to limit the number of embryos transferred to one or two.

Kristin comments:

During my first IVF cycle, we transferred two embryos. This was the standard at our clinic based on my age. When the attempt failed, I was ready to increase the number of embryos transferred to three to increase my chances of getting pregnant. I began another fresh IVF cycle and, when we got close to the transfer, I discussed my desire to transfer three embryos with my RE. He suggested we wait to make the decision based on our embryo quality.

On the day of my transfer, the embryologist refused to transfer more than two embryos because he deemed the two best to be of excellent quality. When I became pregnant with twins, I was extremely thankful that my doctors held their ground and did not let me talk them into transferring more embryos. I had a very difficult pregnancy. If my husband and I decide to try IVF again, we will seriously consider transferring one embryo to reduce my risk of carrying multiples again.

Rebecca comments:

I was on the opposite end of the spectrum as Kristin (see preceding comments). I was weeks away from turning 41 during my first IVF attempt. When we learned that we had six blasts available for transfer, we just assumed that we would transfer two and freeze the rest. Our RE counseled us to transfer all. This was extremely concerning to us, but our RE explained that multiples, especially high order multiples, would be EXTREMELY rare at my age, and that he felt the most aggressive approach (that would also save precious time and money) would be to transfer all. This same office scenario played itself out two more times, until our 3rd, and successful, IVF. For us, it took the transfer of a total of 18, five-day blasts to finally bring our boy/girl twins into this world.

51. How can you have an ectopic pregnancy after IVF?

The exact mechanism responsible for an ectopic pregnancy following an IVF procedure is unknown. Some believe that embryo migration up into the fallopian tubes occurs because of local cellular activity or fluid mechanics present inside the uterus. Sometimes the opening of the fallopian tube in the uterus is dilated because of disease, making it easier for the embryos to enter the tubes.

As described in Part 3, an ectopic pregnancy can occur within the section of the fallopian tube that passes through the muscle of the uterus or within the short segment of fallopian tube that remains after surgical removal of the tube. The incidence of ectopic pregnancy following IVF ranges from 0.5 % to 3%, but this figure may be decreasing. For the past several years, embryo transfer has been routinely performed using ultrasound to properly guide the embryo catheter to the optimal uterine location, which may help to reduce the risk of an ectopic pregnancy. However, even ultrasound guided embryo transfer cannot eliminate the possibility of an ectopic pregnancy after IVF.

The incidence of ectopic pregnancy following IVF ranges from 0.5 % to 3%.

52. Are there age or other restrictions on who should do IVF?

Age restrictions for IVF vary from clinic to clinic. In general, women older than age 40 have a markedly lower chance for a live birth compared with women younger than 40 years old. Age is probably the most important factor influencing the outcome of an IVF cycle. Many clinics will not treat patients older than age 42, and some malpractice carriers dictate that physicians not perform IVF on patients older than 43 years old with their own eggs because of the poor IVF delivery rates related to advancing age.

A woman's chances for successful stimulated IVF can also be predicted by measurement of her FSH and estradiol levels on cycle day 3. Elevations in either hormone are associated with poor IVF success rates, so many clinics impose additional restrictions once the FSH or estradiol levels are known to be elevated. The clomiphene citrate challenge test (CCCT) is another means by which to assess ovarian reserve and predict IVF success. Older women, those with elevated FSH levels on cycle day 3, and those with elevated estradiol levels may consider IVF with donor eggs or adoption.

Natural Cycle IVF has emerged as another treatment alternative for patients with diminished ovarian reserve. Remember that tests of ovarian reserve predict a patient's response to fertility medications but no test exists to predict the presence or absence of a healthy egg in a given patient. The only true means to determine the presence of a healthy egg is delivering of a healthy child—that proves that the patient had at least one good egg! Interestingly, the oldest woman to successfully conceive and deliver a healthy baby with her own egg using IVF was a patient who underwent Natural Cycle IVF and delivered at age 49.

Rebecca comments:

At over 40 years of age, I was fortunate that I had an RE that saw beyond my chronological age and aggressively worked with my husband and me to achieve a pregnancy and live birth using my own eggs. Our third and successful IVF resulted in boy/girl twins from eggs retrieved the day before my 42nd birthday. That said, our family building journey (two IUIs, three IVFs) was not an easy process, nor an inexpensive undertaking. It took an immeasurable amount of commitment on the parts of my husband and me; it was a journey best faced as a strong, unified team. We suffered heartbreaking losses and cycle failures. With each setback we had to regroup, reassess, reevaluate our finances, and discuss our options with our RE. We moved through the medical intervention 'process' gaining an understanding that we took a great deal of emotional and financial risk with every cycle. As we tried to establish realistic expectations from each cycle, we also tried to define the time point or cycle number where we might move on and explore different treatment or family building options. We had a firm belief that it was absurd to bring a child into a family situation that was emotionally and/or financially exhausted. Each patient must face making their own family building decisions, but it is important to consider all the issues (emotional, medical and financial) and enter into discussions with your RE (early and often!), when making decisions to move forward with IVF at advanced maternal age.

53. What is ICSI, and how does it differ from IVF?

In routine IVF, eggs are placed in a laboratory dish in culture media together with prepared sperm. The eggs and sperm are allowed to spontaneously fertilize overnight. The fertilized eggs then develop in the incubator until the embryo transfer procedure, which is usually performed 3 to 5 days after the egg retrieval.

Intracytoplasmic sperm injection (ICSI) differs from IVF in that each egg is individually injected with a

Intracytoplasmic sperm injection (ICSI) differs from IVF in that each egg is individually injected with a single sperm.

single sperm using a tiny needle under microscopic guidance (**Figure 4**). The resulting embryo is then cultured similarly to an embryo produced in a non-ICSI IVF treatment.

ICSI was initially introduced by the IVF team working at the Brussels Free University in Belgium. At that time, assisted fertilization was being attempted through insertion of the sperm under the eggshell (**zona pellucida**). The Belgian group took the extra step of injecting the sperm not only under the eggshell but actually into the middle of the egg itself. The first ICSI pregnancies were reported in 1992. Since then, tens of thousands of children have been born as a result of this unique procedure.

Both ICSI and non-ICSI IVF have similar pregnancy rates and outcomes. The embryos produced by either method should not be considered to be superior to

Zona pellucida

The outer cellular membrane that surrounds the egg and embryo up to the blastocyst stage of development.

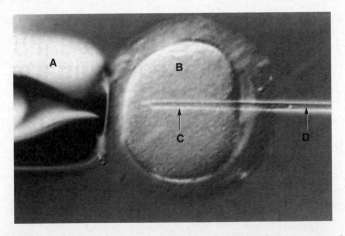

Figure 4   Photography of an actual ICSI being performed in a laboratory. A holding pipette (A) holds the egg (B) in place. Within the ICSI needle (C), the sperm (D) can be seen. The sperm was injected immediately after this photo was taken.

Source: © 2006 American Society for Reproductive Medicine.

those created with the other. ICSI is simply a method to ensure that the egg is fertilized. ICSI is a safe and proven IVF method that does not increase the likelihood that the child conceived in this way will have a birth defect.

54. Who needs ICSI, and how can my reproductive endocrinologist be certain that I need it?

Most couples undergoing treatment with IVF do not require ICSI. The most common indication for ICSI is male factor infertility associated with an abnormal semen analysis. Therefore, men with unproven fertility whose sperm count, motility, or morphology is suboptimal are appropriate candidates for IVF with ICSI to ensure fertilization of the ova.

Another common indication for ICSI is unexplained infertility. In these couples, neither the man nor the woman has any apparent fertility-related problems. Their diagnostic evaluation is entirely normal, yet infertility exists. In such couples, traditional IVF may result in fertilization failure in 20%–40% of IVF cycles. By using ICSI, the eggs are "forced" to fertilize, and the pregnancy rates are usually high. Fertilization rates with ICSI are usually 60%–80% depending upon egg and sperm factors.

55. My husband and I were told by one RE that we needed ICSI, but another RE says that we don't. What should we do?

ICSI is accepted as a standard treatment option for infertile couples with severe male factor infertility. In most clinics, approximately 50% to 90% of the eggs that are injected with sperm using ICSI will fertilize normally.

Approximately 50% to 90% of the eggs that are injected with sperm using ICSI will fertilize normally.

Some eggs do not survive after injection with the sperm and subsequently degenerate.

The criteria regarding what constitutes severe male factor infertility, however, vary from clinic to clinic. Some clinics use ICSI for all (or nearly all) patients based on the theory that assisted fertilization is better than no fertilization at all, but most clinics employ ICSI based upon specific sperm parameters. In general, ICSI is employed in cases where the semen analysis reveals abnormalities related to sperm count (less than 20 million/mL), sperm motility (less than 50% are motile), or sperm morphology (less than 30% have a normal shape). ICSI should also be considered in couples with no previous evidence of fertilization or a history of failed fertilization with a prior IVF attempt. ICSI must be used in cases of sperm obtained from the testicle or epididymis in men with azoospermia (see Question 31). Some clinics use ICSI in all cases of IVF with frozen donor sperm.

Not all cases are clear-cut, for example, in our clinic we often perform an IVF/ICSI split if sperm parameters are normal but the couple has no previous pregnancies. That is, the eggs that are collected during the oocyte retrieval phase are divided between normal fertilization and ICSI. If some component of male factor infertility is present, splitting the eggs between ICSI and IVF may reveal whether the sperm can actually fertilize an egg. If the eggs fail to fertilize with IVF but fertilize normally with ICSI, then the logical conclusion would be that the sperm is incapable of fertilizing the egg with IVF alone. Couples with unexplained fertilization failure with IVF may have a problem with the sperm, the egg, or both. In such cases a repeat cycle of IVF using ICSI will usually yield good fertilization results and, ideally, a pregnancy.

56. What is the Sperm Chromatin Structure Assay (SCSA), and should my husband have it done?

The **Sperm Chromatin Structure Assay (SCSA)** has been proposed as a means to predict the likelihood of pregnancy in cases of male factor infertility. This test analyzes the degree of DNA fragmentation present in a representative sample of sperm. Increased levels of DNA fragmentation seem to be associated with reduced pregnancy rates, including poorer treatment outcomes with IVF and ICSI. There is no level of fragmentation above which pregnancy is completely ruled out, however, so the SCSA cannot ultimately provide a means to absolutely recommend the use of donor sperm over the sperm from the male partner. If a couple is making a choice between the use of donor sperm compared with partner sperm, then the SCSA may provide a relative indication to use the donor sperm option. At this time, most experts consider this test to be experimental.

Sperm Chromatin Structure Assay (SCSA®)

A laboratory test used to determine the degree of DNA fragmentation within a sperm sample.

57. I was told I need assisted hatching. What is this, and why is it done?

Dr. Gordon's older brother, Steven, used to tease him by claiming that he was hatched and not born, but actually all of us do "hatch" in early embryonic life. The human embryo hatches out of the eggshell (zona pellucida) at the blastocyst stage of development. **Assisted hatching** involves weakening the zona to facilitate the emergence of the embryo following its transfer into the uterus after IVF. Proponents of assisted hatching suggest that it increases implantation and pregnancy rates.

Assisted hatching can be performed chemically or, more recently, using a laser. In the chemical technique,

Assisted hatching

The process of making a small hole in the shell (zona pellucida) surrounding the embryo prior to embryo transfer to promote its implantation in the uterus.

a dilute acid solution is used to dissolve the external eggshell. Some clinics still perform mechanical hatching, in which a slit is made in the eggshell. Along with many other clinics, we have moved to laser-assisted hatching, in which a laser is used to thin the zona, sparing the embryo from any exposure to the chemicals used in hatching (see **Figure 5**).

There is some controversy regarding which patients benefit most from assisted hatching, and the indications for assisted hatching remain somewhat unclear. Most clinics recommend this procedure in cases where the female partner is older than age 37, has diminished ovarian reserve with increased levels of FSH, or is undergoing a frozen embryo transfer (FET) with previously cryopreserved embryos. Patients who have previously failed IVF following replacement of good-quality embryos may also benefit from assisted embryo hatching.

The risks of assisted hatching are believed to be quite low. There have been reports of increased rates of

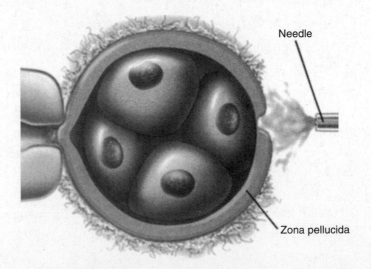

Needle

Zona pellucida

Figure 5   Assisted hatching.

Source: © 1995 Humanatomy® Illustrated

identical twinning following mechanical hatching (but not after chemical- or laser-assisted hatching). There is no evidence that assisted hatching harms the embryo or causes any increased rate of birth defects in children.

Carol comments:

After my first IVF attempt failed for no obvious reason, the RE suggested that we utilize assisted hatching during our second attempt. We immediately moved into a second fresh cycle and employed assisted hatching. From my perspective, there was no difference. The procedure happened after the egg retrieval, so I was not involved. I did get pregnant during the second cycle, and in theory, the assisted hatching was the primary variable that was different.

58. Which types of drug protocols are used in IVF, and how is the most appropriate protocol selected?

Although several drugs and protocols are available to stimulate the ovaries to produce extra eggs for IVF, most clinics utilize only a few of these stimulation protocols. (See **Tables 6, 7**, and **8** for a list of drugs.)

One of the more common IVF protocols is called **luteal suppression** (or long luteal or simply just long) and involves suppression of the ovaries using a GnRH-analog (Lupron) during the luteal phase of the menstrual cycle preceding the planned IVF treatment cycle. Once the ovaries are suppressed, ovarian stimulation is accomplished with daily injections of gonadotropins (e.g., Gonal-F, Follistim). Lupron is usually continued until the day of the HCG trigger shot. A common variation of this protocol is to stop Lupron at the time of starting stimulation. Not surprisingly, this protocol is called "stop Lupron."

Luteal suppression

A stimulation protocol that involves suppression of the pituitary gland and ovary prior to initiating stimulation with fertility medications.

Table 6   Gonadotropin Preparations

Trade Name, Manufacturer	Source
FSH/LSH-containing preparations	
Pergonal, EMD Serono	Urine of menopausal women
Repronex, Ferring	Urine of menopausal women
Menopur, Ferring	Urine of menopausal women
Humegon, Schering-Plough	Urine of menopausal women
FSH-containing preparations	
Bravelle, Ferring	Urine of menopausal women
Fertinex, EMD Serono	Urine of menopausal women
Gonal-F, EMD Serono	Recombinant, Chinese hamster ovary cells
Follistim, Schering-Plough	Recombinant, Chinese hamster ovary cells
LH-only-containing preparation	Recombinant
Luveris, EMD Serono	

FSH, follicle-stimulating hormone; LH, luteinizing hormone.

Table 7   Human Chorionic Gonadotropin Preparations

Trade Name, Manufacturer	Source	Formations
Profasi, EMD Serono	Urine of pregnant females	10,000 IU IM
Pregnyl, Schering-Plough	Urine of pregnant females	10,000 IU IM
Novarel, Ferring	Urine of pregnant females	10,000 IU IM
Chorex, Hyrex	Urine of pregnant females	10,000 IU IM
Ovidrel, EMD Serono	Recombinant, Chinese hamster ovary cells	250 µg SC

Table 8   Gonadotropin-Releasing Hormone Agent Agonist/Antagonist Preparations

Trade Name, Manufacturer	Formulations
Lupron Depot, Abbott	1 mg/0.2 mL = 20 U SC
Synarel, Searle	2 mg/mL intranasal
Zoladex, AstraZeneca	3.6 mg SC
Antagon, Schering-Plough	250 µg/0.5 mL SC
Cetrotide, EMD Serono	250 µg/1 mL SC

Another common protocol is called **flare stimulation**. In this case, the woman does not take any medications until the second day of her menstrual cycle. At that time, a microdose (most commonly) of Lupron is used to "flare" the pituitary gland and induce it to release its store of FSH and LH. Simultaneously, gonadotropins are started, producing a "one–two punch" in terms of ovarian stimulation. Premature ovulation of the eggs rarely occurs despite the low dose of GnRH agonist utilized in this protocol.

A third, more recent option is **GnRH-antagonist** stimulation, in which GnRH antagonists are added later in the stimulation to prevent premature ovulation. In this method, the gonadotropins are started on cycle day 2 of a normal menstrual period. Once the follicles have reached a specific size (usually 12 to 14 mm), the woman begins the GnRH-antagonist medication, which almost instantaneously prevents the pituitary gland from generating an LH surge.

Some reproductive endocrinologists prescribe oral contraceptive pills to their female patients prior to beginning the actual ovarian stimulation drugs, but this practice varies between patients and fertility

Treatment Options: In Vitro Fertilization (IVF)

Flare stimulation protocol

A technique of follicular stimulation that begins at the start of a spontaneous menstrual cycle.

Gonadotropin-releasing hormone (GnRH) antagonist

Medication that quickly interferes with the production of follicle-stimulating hormone and luteinizing hormone by the pituitary gland, preventing premature ovulation during a treatment cycle.

clinics. We have found that the use of birth control pills often results in oversuppression of the ovaries and cycle cancellation except in those patients known to be high responders (women with PCOS, in particular).

The type of protocol selected for any patient (i.e., luteal suppression, flare stimulation or GnRH antagonist) depends on the individual patient and the philosophy of the fertility clinic. Factors that may influence the type of stimulation protocol selected include the patient's age, her day 3 hormone levels, her follicle antral count as determined by ultrasound, and her previous responses to any other attempts at ovarian stimulation.

59. What is Natural-Cycle IVF? And why does my fertility clinic not offer this treatment?

Natural-Cycle IVF (NC-IVF) has been proposed as a means of reducing the risk of multiple pregnancies, eliminating the costs and risks associated with fertility drugs, and reducing the stress and time commitment needed for traditional stimulated IVF. This approach has been espoused by a number of leaders in the field of IVF, including Dr. Robert Edwards, whose pioneering work, along with Dr. Patrick Steptoe's, led to the birth of the world's first IVF baby, Louise Brown, using NC-IVF in 1978.

NC-IVF avoids the use of expensive ovarian stimulation drugs and their associated cost of about $4,000 per treatment cycle. With NC-IVF, the risks of ovarian hyperstimulation, multiple pregnancy, and the issues of cryopreserved extra embryos are avoided as only one embryo is produced. Total cost of NC-IVF is about 20% to 25% of the total cost of a conventional IVF cycle.

However, NC-IVF has its own set of disadvantages. For example, by not using fertility drugs, unexpected premature "LH surging" or ovulation can occur, leading to cancellation of the planned egg retrieval. This occurs in about 10% to 15% of treatment cycles. In such cases, if the fallopian tubes are open, the doctor may recommend converting the treatment to an intrauterine insemination (IUI) cycle. Furthermore, because only one egg and one embryo are produced, the chances for pregnancy are less than with conventional IVF when two or more embryos are transferred. Proponents of NC-IVF expect the "cumulative" pregnancy rate for NC-IVF to be similar to a single cycle of conventional IVF within 1 to 3 treatment cycles of NC-IVF.

The best candidates for NC-IVF are patients with regular menstrual cycles who are less than 36 years old and have normal ovarian reserve. Patients with tubal-factor infertility or male factor infertility may be good candidates for NC-IVF before resorting to conventional IVF. Older patients, patients with previous stimulated cycle IVF failures, patients with poor ovarian reserve or unexplained infertility all can be considered for NC-IVF, but may experience lower pregnancy rates compared with younger patients with well-defined fertility issues and no previous fertility treatments.

Many European fertility centers routinely use NC-IVF with good success rates. For a variety of reasons, the availability of NC-IVF in the United States has been limited. We believe that NC-IVF will soon become increasingly available as patients demand less stressful and less costly fertility treatments that utilize little to no fertility drugs with good pregnancy rates. In our clinic, we have routinely demonstrated pregnancy rates of 25% per successful egg collection and 30%-40% pregnancy rates per embryo transfer with NC-IVF. We have seen success in patients who had previously failed stimulated IVF and were told that donor egg IVF was their only option, so NC-IVF may represent a viable treatment option for many infertile couples—even those with a poor prognosis with stimulated cycle IVF.

60. My reproductive endocrinologist has recommended a protocol that uses birth control pills. Why would birth control pills be used in IVF?

Birth control pills or, more correctly, oral contraceptive pills (OCPs) can be used as a part of the IVF stimulation protocol in several different settings.

First, in patients who are known or suspected to be high responders, OCPs may help mitigate the risk of ovarian hyperstimulation syndrome (OHSS; see Question 63). Second, in patients without predictable regular menstrual cycles, OCPs can be used in combination with Lupron to initiate an IVF cycle. In our practice, we usually start OCPs in such cases after confirming with a blood test that the woman has not recently ovulated. Then, after 1 week on OCPs, we add Lupron. After 1 more week, we stop the OCPs and continue the Lupron and wait for withdrawal bleeding. Once a patient has bled, we begin the gonadotropin stimulation.

Some clinics use OCPs as part of the protocol for microdose Lupron (MDL) flare, traditional flare, or GnRH-antagonist (Antagon, Centrotide) cycles in the hope that pretreatment with OCPs will prevent one follicle from growing faster than the other follicles once the stimulation has begun. We have not routinely used

OCPs with our MDL flare patients, as we have rarely had problems with the emergence of a single dominant follicle compared with the more common problem of oversuppression and a cancelled cycle. Given that prolonged OCP use can lead to oversuppression in low responders, we use these medications very carefully.

Prolonged OCP use can lead to oversuppression in low responders.

61. I had an allergic reaction to the progesterone in oil shots. Does this mean that I cannot do IVF?

Following follicle aspiration, most clinics place patients on progesterone supplementation. The rationale behind the supplemental progesterone is that following egg collection, ovarian hormone production may be impaired because many of the hormone-producing cells are removed at the time of follicle aspiration. In addition, the use of GnRH agonists such as Lupron may diminish ovarian steroid production following egg collection. Progesterone supplementation has evolved over the years to include patients undergoing both stimulated IUI cycles and IVF.

Although many clinics tend to use progesterone-in-oil injections, equivalent pregnancy rates have been reported in patients using only vaginal progesterone supplementation. Allergic reactions to progesterone are infrequent, but switching patients to vaginal progesterone usually resolves the problem.

Another strategy to maintain progesterone production after IUI or egg collection involves the use of HCG booster shots to enhance steroid production from the patient's ovaries rather than relying on an outside source. Unfortunately, the use of HCG boosters may also increase the woman's risk of ovarian hyperstimulation syndrome.

The use of HCG boosters may also increase the woman's risk of ovarian hyperstimulation syndrome.

62. My doctor has prescribed estrogen for me but the package says not to take it if you are pregnant. What should I do?

As noted in earlier questions, the ovary produces both estrogen and progesterone until production of these hormones is taken over by the placenta at approximately 8 to 10 weeks of pregnancy. Estrogen and progesterone are critical hormones for the normal development of the endometrial lining of the uterus. Both medications are frequently used in patients undergoing a frozen embryo transfer (FET) or donor-egg IVF. Estrogen thickens the lining and then progesterone causes the lining to mature, ultimately allowing for the embryo's implantation. Without these hormones, all FET cycles would have to be performed during spontaneous menstrual cycles (see Question 73) and donor-egg IVF would be possible only using frozen embryos, as there would be no way to synchronize the reproductive cycles of the donor and the recipient. There is no evidence that the estrogen used to synchronize these cycles presents any risk to the developing fetus or baby.

If there are no risks, then why do the labels of these medications carry such a strong warning? The labeling is an overreaction to previous experience in the United States with the use of a synthetic estrogen called diethylstilbestrol (DES).

During the 1950s to 1960s, this synthetic estrogen (which is not the natural estrogen used today) was given to women who were threatening to miscarry. Unfortunately, DES did not function in a normal fashion in terms of how it interacted with the estrogen receptors in the cells of the developing female reproductive tract in the unborn daughters of mothers who were prescribed

DES. As a result, many of those women whose mothers took DES during their pregnancy were found to have significant reproductive tract abnormalities. In addition to cervical and uterine abnormalities, they were at a higher risk for an unusual form of vaginal cancer called clear cell carcinoma. Appropriately, DES was taken off the market. At this point in time, the impact of previous DES exposure in the U.S. population has greatly waned as most of the DES daughters have passed beyond child bearing age.

Following the DES debacle, the U.S. government decided that all reproductive steroids should be labeled as being contraindicated in pregnancy. This mandate applies to both progesterone and estrogen compounds. Today, however, the estrogens and progesterones prescribed by fertility physicians are exactly equivalent to the body's own natural estrogen and progesterone produced by the ovary and by the placenta. Women who are prescribed these medications by their physician can take them without any worry that somehow these medications will have an adverse impact on their unborn children.

63. My doctor said that I might get ovarian hyperstimulation syndrome. What is ovarian hyperstimulation syndrome, and what can I do to prevent it?

Ovarian hyperstimulation syndrome (OHSS) is a complication associated with the use of fertility drugs. As the ovarian follicles grow, they secrete a wide range of substances, the most important of which is estrogen. Estrogen causes the lining of the uterus to thicken, enabling the embryo to implant there after ovulation and embryo transfer. Estrogen levels usually directly correlate with the number of growing follicles.

Ovarian hyperstimulation syndrome (OHSS) is a complication associated with the use of fertility drugs.

After a woman receives an HCG injection, her follicles eventually collapse, releasing the eggs within; the follicles may also be aspirated with a needle to harvest the eggs for IVF. Within a few days, the fluid within the follicles is restored. Each follicle is now called a corpus luteum (Latin for "yellow body"), referring to the fact that it contains large stores of cholesterol used to produce the steroid hormones estrogen and progesterone. In addition, the follicle begins to produce a host of other growth factors—including vascular endothelial growth factor (VEGF), a protein that is likely responsible for the emergence of OHSS.

Mild OHSS results in enlarged, tender ovaries but usually only minimal free fluid in the abdominal cavity. By contrast, moderate and severe forms of OHSS are associated with fluid accumulation in the abdominal cavity or sometimes even in the pleural cavity surrounding the lungs. In its severe form, OHSS can result in nausea, vomiting, shortness of breath, and dehydration. As the fluid builds up in the abdomen, the woman becomes increasingly uncomfortable, and diminished blood flow to the kidneys may lead to decreased urine production. This situation can spiral downward rapidly, and complications of blood clot formation and kidney damage can occur if OHSS is left untreated.

Patients with severe OHSS are best managed in the hospital.

Paracentesis

Placement of a needle through the abdominal wall so as to remove excess abdominal fluid.

Patients with severe OHSS are best managed in the hospital, where they can receive intravenous resuscitation and the fluid can be removed via **paracentesis**. Occasionally, the fluid around the lungs may need to be removed if the woman is suffering from respiratory difficulties. However, most of the respiratory complaints associated with OHSS result from the inability of the diaphragm to move appropriately given the marked amount of fluid present within the abdomen. Some clinics manage OHSS by periodically draining the fluid accumulating in the abdomen using a transvaginal aspiration technique similar to an egg collection. Patients usually experience prompt relief, although repeat procedures may be needed if the fluid reaccumulates over the following days.

Prevention of OHSS is always the best strategy. OHSS can best be avoided by judicious use of fertility medications, which is why most physicians individualize gonadotropin doses based on the patient's history, the appearance of her ovaries on ultrasound, and her previous response (if any) to fertility medications. Patients older than age 35 in whom fewer than 12 eggs are retrieved rarely develop significant hyperstimulation. In contrast, patients with polycystic ovarian syndrome are at the highest risk for developing OHSS. Other high-risk patients include women who have many small and medium-size follicles associated with high estrogen levels at the time of HCG administration. However, not all patients who fall into this category will develop OHSS, and some women who might not otherwise seem to be at risk for it will, in fact, go on to develop the syndrome. This randomness of OHSS makes the decision-making process somewhat problematic when trying to prevent this complication.

A woman who exhibits an excessive response to fertility medications associated with a large number of follicles and a high estrogen level should be counseled regarding OHSS prevention strategies. The first option is to withhold the HCG trigger shot, cancel the cycle, and avoid any attempt at pregnancy. Alternatively, a reduced amount of HCG (5,000 units) can be given, followed by follicle aspiration, egg fertilization, and freezing of the embryos with no fresh transfer in that cycle. In such cases, the severe form of hyperstimulation is rarely encountered. In our practice, we have experienced outstanding pregnancy rates during subsequent FET cycles in these patients. Even if no transfer is performed, the woman may still require a brief hospitalization or drainage of abdominal fluid. Ultimately, it is the HCG trigger shot or the HCG produced by a successful pregnancy cycle that induces the ovarian production of VEGF and the other substances that are the cause of OHSS.

In patients who are stimulated without GnRH agonists (Lupron), an alternative method to reduce the risk of hyperstimulation is to use Lupron itself as a trigger rather than HCG. Given that the majority of women undergoing IVF are already taking Lupron, however, this strategy would apply to only a small percentage of the patients pursuing infertility treatment. Furthermore, this strategy would simply eliminate the initial symptoms of OHSS associated with the HCG trigger shot; if pregnancy subsequently occured, the patient would still be at risk for the OHSS associated with a successful cycle.

OHSS is an unpleasant experience for patients, but fortunately the incidence of severe OHSS is low (only 1% to 2%) and the vast majority of patients recover quickly with no long-term problems. In cases where OHSS is associated with pregnancy, this problem can last 2 to 3 weeks and may require several procedures to drain excess fluid. In addition, because of the dehydration associated with severe OHSS, pregnant patients with this syndrome are at risk for the formation of blood clots in the leg or lung. To prevent this complication, most hospitalized patients receive prophylactic daily doses of a blood thinner (**heparin**).

Heparin

An injectable medication that is used to prevent blood clot formation.

64. Why would my doctor suggest IVF if all of my tests are normal?

Upon completion of the diagnostic evaluation, approximately 10% to 15% of couples will be found to have unexplained infertility, meaning that all of their tests are normal. Such couples are probably best called "subfertile," and most can successfully conceive with IVF. Prior to the introduction of IVF, couples with unexplained infertility had a poor chance of achieving pregnancy with other treatment methods. Couples with unexplained infertility can consider IUI with or without fertility drugs prior to attempting IVF, but these treatments are much less successful than IVF. In addition, use of fertility drugs and IUI can be associated with an unacceptable high rate of multiple pregnancy, leaving patients confused about this approach to fertility treatment.

Couples with unexplained infertility can consider IUI with or without fertility drugs prior to attempting IVF.

We do not know precisely why couples with unexplained infertility are infertile. Some evidence suggests that the source of the problem may be tubal dysfunction or sperm–egg interaction. Often, a fertility center uses IVF together with ICSI in such couples to ensure that fertilization of the ova occurs. Today, thanks to these techniques, couples with unexplained infertility have a very strong likelihood of ultimately achieving a successful pregnancy with IVF.

65. What is a blastocyst transfer?

On the third day after egg collection, embryos are referred to as cleavage-stage embryos. At this point, each embryo contains 6 to 10 discrete cells (**blastomeres**). When assessing these embryos for quality, the embryologist grades them based on the number and appearance of the blastomeres. Embryos that have equal-size blastomeres with no fragmentation are usually given a good grade (Grade I), whereas embryos that have extensive

Blastomeres

The individual cells present in an early cleavage-stage embryo.

fragmentation with unequal-size blastomeres are given a poor grade (Grade IV). In general, higher-grade embryos have a much better chance of implanting successfully and generating a pregnancy.

If the embryos are maintained in culture beyond day 3, they first form a solid ball containing approximately 30 to 50 cells, called a **morula**. Over the next day or two, this solid ball of cells becomes a hollow sphere with a clearly defined inner cell mass. This hollow ball of cells is called a blastocyst. Many clinics maintain the embryos in culture until the fifth to seventh day to allow for improved selection of embryos to transfer.

Morula

An early stage of embryonic development in which the embryo consists of a solid ball of cells; the morula is formed prior to the blastocyst.

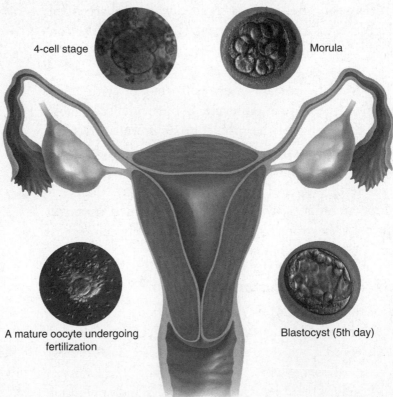

4-cell stage

Morula

A mature oocyte undergoing fertilization

Blastocyst (5th day)

Figure 6   Stages of embryo development.

Source: © 1997 Humanatomy® Illustrated.

Patients who undergo an embryo transfer on day 5 or 6 after egg collection are usually referred to as having a blastocyst transfer although, occasionally, the embryo may actually be at the morula stage of development. (See **Figure 6**.)

66. My clinic performs both day-3 and day-5 embryo transfers, How do they decide which day to do a transfer?

The decision to transfer embryos on day 3 or day 5 is one that requires careful thought. In general, embryos that have formed blastocysts have a better chance of implanting successfully. Unfortunately, not all embryos will progress to the blastocyst stage outside of the body. This fact raises the question as to whether the embryos that fail to form a blastocyst would have initiated a pregnancy if they had been transferred back into the uterus on day 3. Some studies have, indeed, demonstrated acceptable pregnancy rates with day-3 transfers of embryos that were of marginal quality and that, based on historical data, would have been unlikely to form blastocysts in culture. Clearly, the pregnancy rate in the absence of an embryo transfer will be zero, whereas even embryos of borderline quality, if transferred on day 3, may potentially lead to a pregnancy. On the other hand, following normal fertilization inside the fallopian tube, the human embryo does not arrive into the uterus until after day 5 following ovulation. There may be improved synchronization between the embryo and endometrial lining when an embryo transfer is performed on day 5, possibly leading to enhanced implantation rates. Unfortunately, there is no way to do a study in which the exact same embryo is transferred on day 3 and day 5 in order to answer this question.

Patients who undergo an embryo transfer on day 5 or 6 after egg collection are usually referred to as having a blastocyst transfer.

Treatment Options: In Vitro Fertilization (IVF)

So how can you decide between a day-3 and a day-5 embryo transfer? Many clinics make the decision on day 3. If a patient has a certain number of high-quality embryos on day 3, then the embryos are maintained in culture for 2 additional days to allow for further embryo selection at the time of transfer. If the embryos fail to progress to the blastocyst stage, however, then there is no transfer—which often results in profound patient disappointment. If a limited number of embryos are available on day 3 and no embryo selection is needed, then the benefit of a day-5 embryo transfer may be limited to the improved synchronization between embryo and endometrium. In our Natural Cycle IVF program, we have become more and more convinced of the benefit of extended embryo culture. Some marginal-appearing day 3 embryos (4–5 cells) have developed into beautiful blastocysts and led to pregnancy and delivery. Some top grade 8-cell embryos have failed to divide after day 3, resulting in a cancelled embryo transfer. Some patients who failed to conceive with a top quality day-3 embryo have subsequently conceived with a day-5 transfer. The evidence remains anecdotal but very compelling to us and we have now decided to move all Natural Cycle IVF transfers to day 5.

One additional risk of a day-5 transfer is an increased rate of identical twinning. Carrying identical twins (**monozygotic twins**) is considered to be a higher-risk pregnancy than carrying fraternal twins (**dizygotic twins**). Identical twins often share a placenta (**monochorionic twins**) or may even be located within the same pregnancy sac (**monoamniotic twins**). Both of these conditions are associated with increased rates of pregnancy complications. Finally, a clinic's success with embryo cryopreservation following extended culture

Monozygotic twins

Twins arising from a single fertilized egg (also called identical twins).

Dizygotic twins

Twins resulting from the implantation of embryos from two different eggs (also called fraternal twins).

Monochorionic twins

Monozygotic twins who share a single placenta.

Monoamniotic twins

Monochorionic (identical) twins who share a single gestational sac. Carrying monoamniotic twins is considered to be a very high-risk pregnancy.

should also be carefully considered. Although recent advancements with rapid freezing (vitrification) have resulted in excellent survival and pregnancy rates with blastocysts, not all clinics currently employ this technique. We believe that extended culture must go hand in hand with an excellent cryopreservation program in order to maximize patient success.

67. My endometrium is only 6 to 7 millimeters thick. Can I do anything to improve its thickness?

The thickness of the endometrium normally changes throughout the menstrual cycle. During menstruation, the endometrium is shed. Under the influence of the hormone estradiol, the endometrium then regenerates and usually develops to a normal thickness of 8 or more millimeters (mm). When a woman is undergoing infertility treatment, the thickness of her endometrium is regularly measured using ultrasonography.

When the endometrium fails to develop to at least 8 mm, the embryo may fail to implant because of endometrial immaturity or dyssynchrony. Although this problem is not very common, when it occurs, it can be difficult to correct. Typical treatments consist of providing additional estrogen early in the menstrual cycle or altering the timing of progesterone administration. Other therapeutic agents include small doses of aspirin (80 to 100 mg per day), and some physicians have prescribed sildenafil (Viagra) vaginal suppositories for their female patients with variable success. Some women cannot achieve pregnancy in a fresh IVF embryo transfer cycle but readily become pregnant when the embryos are transferred in a frozen–thawed nonstimulated treatment cycle. On rare occasions, a couple may need to use a gestational carrier to successfully overcome abnormalities involving the endometrium and implantation.

Of course, failure of the endometrium to achieve a minimum thickness of 8 mm does not necessarily translate into a problem with the endometrium. In our practice, we have seen many patients with maximal endometrial development of only 4 to 7 mm successfully achieve pregnancy, including delivery of twins. A variety of testing methods to assess endometrial maturity have been proposed, including endometrial biopsy testing for surface proteins called integrins, but such testing remains somewhat controversial in terms of its predictive value.

68. What are PGD and PGS?

Preimplantation genetic diagnosis (PGD) and **preimplantation genetic screening (PGS)** are techniques that provide diagnostic information concerning an embryo prior to its transfer to the uterus. The vast majority of PGD and PGS procedures are performed by removing 1 or 2 cells (or blastomeres) of a 6- to 8-cell embryo on day 3 of embryo culture following IVF. These cells are rapidly analyzed, and, on day 5, the unaffected embryos are selected for embryo transfer.

PGD was first performed in 1989 in an effort to avoid the transfer of embryos that carried serious genetic disorders (e.g., cystic fibrosis). Thus, couples who undergo PGD do not have infertility but rather are at risk for passing a genetic disease to their children. A wide range of single-gene and chromosomal disorders can now be diagnosed with PGD, including **autosomal recessive diseases** (e.g., cystic fibrosis), **X-linked recessive diseases** (e.g., hemophilia, Duchenne muscular dystrophy), **autosomal dominant diseases** (e.g.,

Preimplantation genetic screening (PGS)

An evaluation that is similar to preimplantation genetic diagnosis but is used to screen embryos in fertility patients for aneuploidy instead of a specific genetic disease.

Couples who undergo PGD do not have infertility but rather are at risk for passing a genetic disease to their children.

Autosomal recessive diseases

Genetic diseases carried on a chromosome other than the X or Y chromosomes (sex chromosomes), in which two abnormal copies of the gene are necessary for the disease to be present.

Huntington's disease), and chromosomal rearrangements (e.g., **balanced translocations**).

PGS is similar to PGD, but refers to screening of embryos produced in the course of fertility treatments. Thus, couples who undergo PGS include infertile patients without an underlying genetic problem. PGS is performed in an attempt to identify those embryos that are genetically abnormal so that improved embryo selection will—ideally—result in improved pregnancy rates and lower miscarriage rates.

69. How safe is PGD or PGS?

An estimated 5,000 cycles of PGD/PGS are being performed in the United States each year. Although the use of these techniques has increased over the past decade, the number of PGD/PGS cycles continues to represent only a small fraction of the more than 100,000 IVF procedures performed annually in the United States alone. The rate of congenital anomalies and of pregnancy complications following PGD/PGS does not appear to be increased over the baseline measurements.

On occasion, misdiagnosis may occur, so patients undergoing PGD/PGS are usually offered traditional prenatal diagnostic tests (chorionic villus sampling-CVS or amniocentesis) to confirm the results. The rates of misdiagnosis in PGD range from 1% to 9%. Embryos from which no diagnostic information is obtained are usually discarded rather than risk embryo transfer, although this policy varies from clinic to clinic. The other risks of PGD/PGS are the same as those associated with any cycle of IVF, including multiple pregnancy and OHSS.

Treatment Options: In Vitro Fertilization (IVF)

X-linked recessive disease

A genetic disease associated with a mutation on the X chromosome. A male carrying such a mutation will have the disorder because he has only one X chromosome, but a female carrying a mutation on just one X chromosome has a normal gene on the other chromosome and so will not be affected by the disease.

Autosomal dominant diseases

Genetic diseases carried on a chromosome other than the X or Y chromosomes (sex chromosomes), in which a single abnormal copy of the gene leads to the presence of the disease.

Balanced translocation

A chromosomal rearrangement in which two chromosomes break apart and re-form as a new chromosome containing parts of both of the original chromosomes.

70. Can PGS improve outcomes after IVF?

PGS has been promoted as a means to improve the odds of a successful IVF cycle. However, a large-scale, randomized, controlled study performed in women older than age 37 failed to demonstrate an improvement in clinical outcome following its use. Although the use of PGS will likely decrease the rate of miscarriage resulting from **aneuploidy**, the overall delivery rate per IVF cycle initiated may not be increased with this technology.

One limitation of PGS is that many embryos at the 6- to 8-cell stage of development are mosaics, meaning that some of these cells carry a normal complement of **chromosomes** while other cells are abnormal. During further embryonic development, the abnormal cells presumably end up relegated to the placenta while the normal cells produce a healthy embryo. The high rate of **mosaicism** in cleavage-stage embryos raises a real concern about the accuracy of PGS. One respected geneticist has estimated a rate of misdiagnosis to be 20% with PGS. Approximately 17% of the time, a normal embryo is incorrectly labeled as abnormal and discarded. Even more concerning is the 3% chance that an abnormal embryo will be labeled normal and then transferred to the uterus.

In the case of couples for whom the use of prenatal diagnosis and possible pregnancy termination are not an option, PGS may be appropriate. According to an October 2006 monograph produced by the European Society of Human Reproduction and Embryology (ESHRE), "Although widely used, PGS is still considered as an experimental procedure, and its clinical utility is not fully proven."

In 2007, the ASRM and SART issued a joint statement concerning the use of PGS (and PGD) saying that there

Aneuploidy

Having an abnormal number of chromosomes.

Many embryos at the 6- to 8-cell stage of development are mosaics.

Chromosomes

One of the threadlike "packages" of genes and other DNA in the nucleus of a cell. Humans have 23 pairs of chromosomes, for a total of 46 in all: 44 autosomes and 2 sex chromosomes.

Mosaicism

The presence of both genetically normal and abnormal cells within an embryo prior to implantation.

is insufficient evidence to support the widespread application of PGS given its failure to improve live birth rates.

(Reprinted with permission of Elsevier from Preimplantation genetic testing: a Practice Committee opinion. The Practice Committee of the Society for Assisted Reproductive Technology, Practice Committee of the American Society for Reproductive Medicine. Fertil Steril 90(5): S136–S143 (November 2008).)

Recommendations: PGD

- Before PGD is performed, genetic counseling must be provided to ensure that patients fully understand the risk for having an affected child, the impact of the disease on an affected child, and the limitations of available options that may help to avoid the birth of an affected child.
- PGD can reduce the risk for conceiving a child with a genetic abnormality carried by one or both parents if that abnormality can be identified with tests performed on a single cell.
- Prenatal diagnostic testing to confirm the results of PGD is encouraged strongly because the methods used for PGD have technical limitations that include the possibility for a false negative result.

Recommendations: PGS

- Before PGS is performed, thorough education and counseling must be provided to ensure that patients fully understand the limitations of the technique, the risk of error, and the lack of evidence that PGS improves live birth rates.
- Available evidence does not support the use of PGS as currently performed to improve live birth rates in patients with advanced maternal age.

- Available evidence does not support the use of PGS as currently performed to improve live birth rates in patients with previous implantation failure.
- Because the prevalence of aneuploidy is high in the embryos of patients with recurrent implantation failure, decisions concerning future treatment should not be based on the results of PGS in one or more cycles.
- Available evidence does not support the use of PGS as currently performed to improve live birth rates in patients with recurrent pregnancy loss.
- Available evidence does not support the use of PGS as currently performed to reduce miscarriage rates in patients with recurrent pregnancy loss related to aneuploidy.

71. What is embryo freezing, and how successful is it?

On the day of embryo transfer, a couple may learn that they have additional embryos of good quality in addition to those embryos that have been selected for embryo transfer. These embryos can be cryopreserved by freezing them in liquid nitrogen. Through a series of carefully orchestrated steps, the embryos are ultimately frozen at a temperature of −196 °C, leaving them in a state of suspended animation in which they can remain for many years. Embryos that have been stored for more than 10 years have successfully generated pregnancies (although most patients tend to use their frozen embryos within 3 to 5 years after they are produced). The pregnancy rates associated with replacing frozen embryos depend on the age of the patient and the quality of the embryos at the time of cryopreservation. Top-quality embryos from young patients may yield pregnancy rates in excess of 50%, whereas poor-quality embryos may not even survive the thawing process. In some clinics, more than 75%

In some clinics, more than 75% of embryos survive the freeze–thaw cycle.

of embryos survive the freeze–thaw cycle. Currently, two methods are used to freeze embryos: "slow cooling" and vitrification. More information on vitrification can be found in Question 72.

Many couples are concerned about their moral obligations concerning their frozen embryos. In such cases, couples may elect to defer embryo freezing, choose to alter their stimulation or pursue Natural Cycle IVF so as to avoid this problem of excess embryos. Extra embryos that are not used to initiate a pregnancy could represent a source of embryonic stem cells. This potential use of extra embryos lies at the heart of the recent political debate in the United States regarding government funding of stem cell research. Clearly, patients should carefully consider the implications of excess frozen embryos as they embark on an IVF cycle. However, not all patients will have extra embryos of high enough quality to be considered for embryo cryopreservation.

Rebecca comments:

I had gone through stim and egg retrieval for my third (and likely last) IVF with my own eggs; egg retrieval occurred the day before my 42nd birthday. I had always responded well to the gonadotropins, and this cycle was no different. I believe my estrogen levels had gone over 10,000 prior to HCG trigger, putting me at risk for developing Ovarian Hyper Stimulation Syndrome (OHSS). On embryo transfer day, I went into the RE's office feeling very bloated and uncomfortable. I knew embryo transfer was going to be very difficult. My RE immediately suspected OHSS and began discussing the option of embryo cryopreservation to allow for frozen embryo transfer (FET) at a later date. I was heartbroken. I knew that I couldn't transfer, but was convinced that my 'older' embryos would suffer from the freezing process. My RE reassured me that my embryos would be frozen using vitrification and that the clinic was seeing freeze/thaw success rates as high as 85%.

I now believe that cryopreservation and FET were the tickets to our success. The FET cycle was the most relaxed cycle I had been through. There were no shots, there was very limited monitoring and blood draws, and my body wasn't being overwhelmed by hormones. On the day of transfer, my embryos were thawed with a 100% freeze/ thaw success rate. The transfer of six blasts was the most comfortable transfer of the three transfers I had been through. Two weeks later I received my BFP (positive beta-HCG) and 8 months later I gave birth to my girl/boy twins. I went from being highly skeptical about cryopreservation to becoming a firm believer in the benefits of this wonderful treatment option.

72. What is vitrification?

For many years, all embryos were frozen using what is known as a slow-cooling protocol. The embryos were placed into a specific solution containing cryoprotectants and the temperature was slowly dropped (−0.33 °C/min) in a very precise manner. Slow-cooling worked best for cleavage stage embryos or embryos frozen on the day after egg collection (2 pn stage). Slow-cooling was not as effective when freezing unfertilized eggs or embryos at the blastocyst stage of development.

Vitrification literally means "turning to glass" and is an ultra-rapid form of cryopreservation (−20,000 °C/min) that basically consists of plunging the egg/embryo into liquid nitrogen resulting in near instantaneous freezing of the egg/embryo. Recovery rates and pregnancy rates have been shown to be superior when vitrification is compared with slow-cooling of eggs and blastocyst stage embryos. Not all clinics currently offer vitrification, but it seems likely that this approach will become the standard method of cryopreservation over the next 5 years.

Since adopting vitrification in April 2007 at Dominion Fertility, our frozen-thaw embryo transfer pregnancy rates are now equivalent to our fresh embryo transfer pregnancy rates. We have abandoned the slow-cooling approach and use vitrification exclusively for our embryo cryopreservation program. Furthermore, many studies have demonstrated remarkable success in the area of egg (oocyte) cryopreservation. Success with freezing unfertilized eggs may offer new hope to cancer patients and to women considering freezing their eggs for future use. In addition, oocyte cryopreservation may allow for the development of oocyte banks similar to sperm banks.

73. What is the difference between a Natural-Cycle frozen embryo transfer (FET) and a medicated FET?

There are two possible options for performing a frozen embryo transfer (FET): Natural-Cycle FET (NC-FET) and medicated FET.

Natural Cycle FET is available to women with regular ovulation and monthly menstrual cycles. In patients with predictable menstrual cycles, we can carefully monitor the cycle to determine the precise timing of ovulation. Alternatively, ovulation can be induced with the administration of an HCG injection. Once the precise date of ovulation is set, then the uterine lining should be receptive to embryo transfer 5 days later (for embryos frozen on day 5 in a previous IVF cycle). In this way, the embryos can be replaced at approximately the time when they would normally be arriving in the uterus.

One problem with Natural-Cycle FET is that the optimal time for implantation may fall at an unpredictable time during the laboratory work schedule, so some clinics choose not to offer NC-FET. In addition, NC-FET demands frequent patient monitoring around the time of ovulation. If a cycle is suboptimal in terms of the estrogen level and endometrial development, then the embryos should not be thawed and the cycle should be cancelled.

A medicated FET allows the couple to avoid some of the pitfalls associated with a NC-FET.

A medicated FET allows the couple to avoid some of the pitfalls associated with a NC-FET. In this type of FET, estrogen pills, shots, or patches are used to prepare the endometrium for embryo implantation. Three days prior to embryo transfer, the woman begins taking progesterone to modify the endometrial lining so that it will be receptive when the embryos are placed. Some clinics prescribe GnRH agonists (such as Lupron) to their patients the month prior to a medicated FET cycle so as to reduce the chances of spontaneous ovulation. The use of Lupron reduces the chances of cycle cancellation owing to unexpected ovulation to near zero.

The choice of estrogen supplementation varies somewhat between clinics. Some clinics prescribe oral estrogens; other clinics administer intramuscular estrogen shots twice a week, and still other clinics use transdermal estrogen patches twice a week. The choice of estrogen protocol is clinic-specific and should be discussed with your reproductive endocrinologist. Many clinics prescribe progesterone-in-oil injections to prepare the lining for embryo transfer. Women who have a progesterone allergy can use progesterone suppositories instead.

Pregnancy rates have not been shown to differ significantly between NC-FET and medicated FET. However, medicated FETs do allow for advance scheduling, which both patients and physicians find attractive. The advantages of NC-FET are its simplicity with no injections (besides the HCG trigger shot) and minimal additional medications with an overall cost savings compared with a medicated FET.

74. My last IVF failed. Should I try again?

To make the best decision about whether to do another IVF, your first step is usually to sit down with your doctor and review your history and the details of the failed cycle. This would include a discussion of the rationale behind attempting IVF in the first place and a careful examination of the results of the IVF cycle. Clearly, if a woman can conceive only through the use of IVF (for example, because she has no fallopian tubes or because her partner's sperm is of such poor quality that no other alternative is available), then the decision becomes one of whether another attempted IVF is warranted.

In reviewing the previous IVF cycle, the woman's response to the stimulation protocol, as well as the findings at the time of egg collection should be carefully examined. If the eggs appeared immature at the time of egg collection, then in the future, the trigger shot should probably be withheld until the follicles reach a larger diameter. If the stimulation and number of eggs are appropriate but fertilization was unexpectedly poor, then the use of ICSI for a future IVF cycle could be considered. If stimulation, fertilization, and embryo development were good and yet the cycle still failed, then consideration should be given to either an FET cycle (if appropriate) or a repeat cycle of IVF. If the stimulation was poor and the number of eggs was suboptimal, then other stimulation protocols should be discussed. If maximum doses were used and a poor response was still seen, then Stimulated Cycle IVF may not be an appropriate choice. In such a case, other options—ranging from Natural Cycle IVF to IUI to donor egg or adoption—may warrant discussion.

In cases where patients have frozen embryos remaining from the fresh IVF, we usually encourage them to attempt pregnancy with a frozen embryo transfer. Many patients who fail to conceive on a fresh IVF will conceive on the FET.

Many patients who fail to conceive on a fresh IVF will conceive on the FET.

The post-IVF consultation is one of the most useful discussions that a couple can have with the physician. It allows the couple to review all aspects of their care and to determine whether IVF represents the best approach to their particular situation. We firmly believe that this feedback is crucial to develop an appropriate plan of treatment for each couple.

Kristin comments:

Obviously, this is a very personal decision that is based on your own emotional, physical, and financial situation. For us, the answer was easy: Yes! At our post-cycle consult with the RE, he reassured us that IVF could work for us. We discussed the quality of our remaining frozen embryos and the chances of conceiving through a FET and ultimately decided to pursue another fresh IVF cycle. We jumped right back into IVF, doing two back-to-back fresh cycles. They were not easy months, emotionally or physically. I had wonderful support from family and friends, and this helped to keep me focused on my ultimate goal of creating a family with

*my husband. I believe it is very important to have some-
body to discuss your fears, concerns, and frustrations with
while cycling, be it an online buddy, family member,
friend, or professional counselor. So often the focus is on the
financial and physical ramifications of IVF, but the emotional toll is often the worst.*

75. When can I do a home pregnancy test after IVF?

In the laboratory we can test for the presence of pregnancy by measuring the level of beta-HCG in either
the urine or the blood. Both types of tests are reliable
and highly accurate, but home pregnancy testing can
yield both false positives and false negatives if performed too early. Performing a pregnancy test within
7 days after the egg collection procedure can result in a
false positive result because of residual HCG after the
shot is given to trigger the final maturation of the
eggs. In addition, the urine pregnancy test may be spu-
riously negative if performed less than 14 days after
the embryo transfer. In our practice, we have had
patients with a serum beta-HCG level of more than
200 mIU/mL who nevertheless had a negative urine
pregnancy test.

We advise patients to obtain a blood pregnancy test 12
to 14 days after an IVF embryo transfer and to avoid
home pregnancy testing. In-office blood pregnancy
tests provide the most reliable and accurate result.

Kristin comments:

*Our RE highly encouraged us to wait for the blood test,
and my husband was extremely adamant that I not do a
home pregnancy test. He did not want me to be given false*

*We advise
patients to
obtain a blood
pregnancy test
12 to 14 days
after an IVF
embryo
transfer and to
avoid home
pregnancy
testing.*

hope by a positive home pregnancy test that turned out not to be a viable pregnancy. The 2-week wait was extremely difficult, but we kept ourselves busy by planning a 5-day trip in the middle of it.

I am really glad I did not do a home pregnancy test with our first IVF because it probably would have been positive, despite the outcome of a chemical pregnancy. To have the hope of pregnancy erased the next day by a low beta would have been more than I could handle emotionally at the time. On our second IVF attempt, I waited until I got the positive beta from the RE, and then I took many home pregnancy tests so I could see that double line for myself.

76. When I went in for my first ultrasound after IVF, my RE saw two gestational sacs at 6.5 weeks, but only one had a fetal pole with a heartbeat. What will happen to the other pregnancy sac?

Such events are not uncommon following IVF. The incidence of a clinical twin pregnancy after IVF is 10% to 33%, with the exact likelihood depending on the number of embryos transferred and the age of the patient. In 30% to 40% of these pregnancies, one gestational sac will be empty, a situation called a blighted ovum pregnancy. Often, these pregnancies will simply disappear. At other times, the woman may experience cramping and bleeding. In such a case, there is a 40% to 50% risk that the healthy gestational sac and fetus will also abort. There is no way to predict the outcome, and there is no medical intervention that can be implemented to preserve the normal sac and fetus. During this difficult time, patients are well advised to rest and decrease their stress as much as possible. Supplemental progesterone may help quiet uterine contractions, but it is not curative.

In women who suffer a twin early pregnancy loss, a medical investigation may be indicated to search for any causes that may have contributed to the early pregnancy loss. Unfortunately, such evaluations may not produce any definitive answers (see Questions 92–99).

Carol comments:

During my first pregnancy, I lost a twin at 8 weeks after fetal cardiac activity was visualized. I do recall a severe episode of cramping, but there was no bleeding involved. In addition to my RE, the other medical professionals involved confirmed that no intervention was necessary. I went on to enjoy a very normal pregnancy and delivered my son at 40.5 weeks.

77. What do the beta-HCG levels mean and what does it mean if my levels don't double every 2 days?

In a normal early pregnancy, regardless of the method of conception, a woman's serum beta-HCG levels will roughly double every 48 hours. Failure of the beta-HCG levels to double may suggest an abnormal intrauterine pregnancy or an ectopic pregnancy. Given that biologic variation can occur in both normal and abnormal pregnancies, however, we cannot assume that a pregnancy is in jeopardy simply because the beta-HCG levels fail to perfectly double. It is estimated that in 15% of normal pregnancies the beta-HCG levels fail to rise in a linear fashion and that in 15% of ectopic pregnancies the beta-HCG rise is completely normal.

In any pregnancy associated with a suboptimal rise in beta-HCG, the outcome can range from a normal intrauterine pregnancy to an abnormal intrauterine

Failure of the beta-HCG levels to double may suggest an abnormal intrauterine pregnancy or an ectopic pregnancy.

pregnancy, and to an ectopic pregnancy. This determination can be made only by performing a transvaginal ultrasound examination. Even then, the sonogram results may be inconclusive. In our practice, we have seen several cases in which patients had abnormal beta-HCG rises and a first sonogram that suggested an early blighted ovum pregnancy, only to discover later that the pregnancy was completely normal.

A common cause for non-linear increases in the beta-HCG level is multiple pregnancy. When patients undergo transfer of two or more embryos, a multiple gestational pregnancy may occur. In roughly 40% of these pregnancies, spontaneous fetal reduction of the extra implanted sacs occurs, resulting in a sudden drop in the beta-HCG level. Initially this decrease might be falsely interpreted as an apparent problem with the pregnancy when, in fact, one surviving embryo is completely healthy. For all these reasons, the blood beta-HCG doubling effect must be viewed as a guide, and not independently predictive of the outcome of any pregnancy.

78. I have recently been diagnosed with cancer. Do I have any options to preserve my fertility?

Treatment and survival rates of cancer are always the first focus of concern when treating cancer patients. But cancer survivors are now living longer and quality of life after treatment including the possibility of fertility should be considered.

There are several fertility treatment options available for the patient recently diagnosed with cancer. In patients with a male partner, IVF can be performed, embryos produced, cryopreserved and later transferred with excellent success rates. The entire IVF stimulation and egg retrieval process can be completed within 2–3 weeks. For single women or women without a male partner, IVF with donor sperm to produce embryos for storage is an option; or they could consider egg cryopreservation (see Question 79). We believe that egg cryopreservation will soon become a routine procedure in the advanced reproductive technologies and especially so for cancer patients.

Finally, some cancer patients have achieved successful pregnancies after later transplantation of their cryopreserved ovarian tissue. In this technique, ovarian tissue is surgically removed prior to chemotherapy or radiation therapy, banked and stored for later autotransplantation in a second surgical procedure. Obviously, egg and embryo cryopreservation have the advantage of avoiding surgery.

For additional information concerning fertility and cancer, we recommend the book *100 Questions and Answers about Fertility and Cancer* by Dr. Kutluk Oktay, Lindsay Beck and Joyce Reincecke.

79. Should I freeze my eggs now so that I can use them in the future?

Recent advances in egg (oocyte) and embryo cryopreservation have radically changed our approach to this topic. It is our belief that egg freezing is now a viable option for fertility preservation.

Until recently, high costs ($10,000–$15,000 per treatment), and very low pregnancy rates (<5% live birth rates) made egg freezing experimental and clinically unacceptable for most patients. With the use of "vitrification" (see Question 72), egg survival, fertilization and pregnancy rates have vastly improved. Currently, the ASRM considers egg freezing to be experimental, but the European Society for Human Reproduction (ESHRE) and many other reputable medical societies do not. Based upon published papers and conference abstracts, especially over the last 3 years, we believe that egg freezing is no longer just a "backup" experimental procedure, but rather it represents another constituent option among the advanced reproductive technologies for women wishing to preserve their fertility.

It is well established that a woman's fertility peaks in her 20s and begins to decline at age 30 with a rapid decline after age 35. Egg quality is directly related to age. Understanding that many women will delay childbirth until they are in their mid to late 30s (or even later) for social, career or economic reasons, it would be logical for these women to consider egg freezing and storing in their 20s or early 30s when their egg quality is at its peak biologic potential. This would allow them a later reproductive option should they experience age-related infertility.

Egg cryopreservation involves the same steps in a stimulated IVF treatment. The patient takes gonadotropin injections for about 7 to 10 days to induce the development of multiple follicles. The eggs are then collected and immediately cryopreserved using "vitrification." Theoretically, the eggs can be stored indefinitely for later fertilization and embryo transfer. We recommend egg cryopreservation only at IVF centers with a proven track record of success with embryo or egg cryopreservation using vitrification, which is a relatively new extension of the advanced reproductive technologies.

PART NINE

Treatment Options: Third-Party Reproduction

How is donor-egg IVF performed?

Where do egg donors come from, and why would a woman want to be a donor?

What screening tests are performed on egg donors?

More . . .

80. Why does my reproductive endocrinologist think that I need to use an egg donor?

Egg donation is a very successful fertility treatment and is usually recommended based upon a woman's age or her previous experience with fertility treatments. Unlike men who are constantly producing new sperm, a woman is born with all of her eggs and is incapable of making more over the course of her lifetime. After the age of 30, fertility begins to decline—markedly so after the age of 35. By age 40, most women will experience infertility. Fertility medications can induce the continued growth of follicles that were initially destined to undergo atresia, allowing patients to undergo treatments with multiple eggs/embryos. However, these drugs will not improve egg quality, as they can only increase the egg quantity.

Egg quantity can be predicted, to a limited degree, by obtaining blood hormone levels for FSH and estradiol on cycle day 3. Elevations in either hormone suggest diminished ovarian reserve. Another test for ovarian reserve is the clomiphene citrate challenge test (CCCT), a simple blood test that measures FSH and estradiol before and after the woman takes Clomid. Many reproductive endocrinologists perform an ovarian transvaginal ultrasound examination and a follicle count to further assess ovarian function. Antimullerian hormone (AMH) is a newer blood test that can be used to predict a patient's response to fertility medications (see Question 10). Women with normal ovarian reserve testing (FSH/estradiol, AMH, antral follicle count, etc.) may rarely demonstrate a low response to fertility medications whereas those with poor ovarian reserve testing almost always have a disappointing stimulation.

When a woman's response to fertility medication is poor, or when she has failed to conceive with previous attempts at IVF or other treatments, or when she has diminished ovarian reserve, then IVF using donor eggs is an excellent option. Since 1984, egg donation has been a cornerstone in treating patients whose egg quality/ quantity have deteriorated, making stimulated IVF a poor choice. By using donated eggs from a woman in her twenties, the infertile patient essentially restores her fertility potential to that of the age of her egg donor. Similarly, the miscarriage rate drops from more than 50% for patients older than age 40 to 10% to 12% with the use of donor eggs.

Since 1984, egg donation has been a cornerstone in treating patients whose egg quality/ quantity have deteriorated.

Egg donation has been used extensively in patients who are perimenopausal or even menopausal. Most clinics have an age restriction in terms of their egg donor recipients, with the most common cut-off age being 50 years old. Unlike the eggs, the uterus slowly ages and remains receptive to implantation (as long as the endometrium is successfully prepared with hormones) well into a woman's fifth and possibly sixth decades of life.

81. How is donor-egg IVF performed?

During a cycle of donor-egg IVF, the egg donor, usually a young healthy woman in her 20s, undergoes a cycle of ovarian stimulation culminating in an egg collection. The eggs are then fertilized with the sperm of the egg donor recipient's partner and the embryos are ultimately transferred into the uterus of the recipient. Most donor-egg IVF arrangements are anonymous, although known donor-egg IVF is possible. In the latter case, the known donor is usually a family member or friend. In our experience, most of our patients prefer to use an anonymous egg donor to avoid family and interpersonal conflicts.

Treatment Options: Third-Party Reproduction

Most medical practices recruit egg donors for their patients, but third-party agencies are also available that act as brokers. The American Society of Reproductive Medicine (ASRM) has developed a set of egg donor screening guidelines, which most practices utilize for screening donors. The guidelines encompass comprehensive screening for infectious and genetic diseases, physical examination, and psychological testing. Since May 2005, the U.S. Food and Drug Administration (FDA) has mandated extensive infectious disease testing in screening all anonymous egg and sperm donors.

The actual treatment cycle for donor-egg IVF essentially combines a fresh IVF cycle (the donor) and a medicated FET cycle (the recipient). The two treatment cycles are synchronized by using GnRH analogs. Usually, the recipient begins estrogen therapy 5 days prior to the start of the egg donor's stimulation so as to provide an adequate time frame for the recipient's endometrium to grow and thicken. After 10 to 14 days of stimulation, the donor receives an injection of HCG (Pregnyl, Profasi, Ovidrel, Novaryl) to mature her eggs. On the same day, the recipient starts progesterone therapy to create a receptive endometrium.

Because most egg donors are young, they tend to respond very well to the ovarian stimulation drugs, producing many high-quality eggs and embryos. Implantation rates with these embryos are also very high, so that usually only one or two embryos are transferred to the recipient. Pregnancy rates usually exceed 50% per initiated cycle, making donor-egg IVF the most successful therapy currently available for infertile couples. Usually, extra embryos that were not transferred can be frozen and stored for later transfer, with excellent pregnancy rates achieved in subsequent conception attempts.

Pregnancy rates usually exceed 50% per initiated cycle of donor-egg IVF.

Donor-egg IVF can be very expensive and is frequently specifically excluded from the list of treatments covered by insurance. Donors often receive compensation of $5,000–$10,000 per completed cycle. When one includes the cost of fertility medications ($4,000), the cost of donor screening (genetic, infectious disease, psychological) and the clinical procedures performed then the total cost can approach $25,000–$30,000.

82. Where do egg donors come from, and why would a woman want to be a donor?

The typical egg donor is a healthy young woman in her twenties who desires to help others in having a baby. In our experience, egg donors tend to be intelligent, altruistic, sincere women who are knowledgeable about the difficulties that many couples face with their infertility. Most egg donors come from the local community near the infertility practice. They have learned about infertility from their friends, family, the Internet, and the media. Many egg donors have their own children and wish to help others to experience parenthood/pregnancy. Other donors state that they are 100% sure that they themselves do not desire children and wish their eggs to be used by someone else who feels differently. Finally, some donors have undergone abortions for unwanted pregnancy and view the egg donation process as a means to work through their ambivalence about that previous decision.

Most of the donors whom we recruit for our practice have a college degree or are actively pursuing one. Most anonymous donors are reimbursed for their time and the expenses involved in the screening and treatment process. The screening usually takes 2 to 3 months to complete and the IVF treatment takes 4 to 6 weeks.

In our experience, women who donate their eggs are very responsible individuals and genuinely concerned about carefully completing their role in the IVF treatment process to achieve a successful outcome.

83. What screening tests are performed on egg donors?

Both the ASRM and the FDA have issued clear screening guidelines and regulations for egg and sperm donors; the guidelines are available on these organizations' respective websites. A typical egg donor evaluation involves a comprehensive history of the donor's health and of her family. A physical examination and comprehensive laboratory screening tests for communicable diseases are also performed. Many centers add genetic testing of the donors. A psychological assessment of all ova donors is routinely performed.

Although the anonymous donor's anonymity is preserved, the results of his or her laboratory tests, psychological profile, physical characteristics, and historical information are shared with the recipient. This information allows recipients to carefully choose their donor and provides a certain level of comfort in knowing that proper screening was performed. Some clinics provide adult photos of their donors, but in our practice we have limited photos to those from childhood to preserve the donors' anonymity.

84. What is a gestational carrier, and when should you consider using one?

A gestational carrier is a woman who has agreed to carry a pregnancy for another woman/couple because the latter has been determined to have medical issues that make a successful pregnancy extremely unlikely or dangerous. A gestational carrier shares no genetic information with the baby she is carrying since the baby is the product of IVF using the eggs/sperm of the genetic parents. Traditional surrogacy (illegal in several states) differs from gestational surrogacy in that the egg is actually produced by the birth mother and pregnancy occurs following insemination in most cases.

Many medical conditions necessitate the use of a gestational carrier, including the absence of a uterus in the would-be mother, either because of a congenital (at birth) condition or when a disease necessitated its surgical removal. A gestational carrier may also be the best option when a woman has a systemic disease that may affect either her own or her baby's health, such as advanced heart disease, severe diabetes, or multiple sclerosis. Likewise, a woman with a history of poor pregnancy outcome—including repetitive pregnancy losses, preterm labor, **incompetent cervix**, or severe **preeclampsia**—may be a good candidate for IVF using a gestational carrier.

Prior to any IVF treatment, thorough screening of the gestational carrier is routinely performed following ASRM guidelines. Gestational carriers are usually well known to the couple and may be relatives or friends. In addition, there are agencies that introduce gestational carriers to prospective patients. In such arrangements, the gestational carrier is usually compensated for her time and energy (especially if the pregnancy proves successful).

When using a gestational carrier, IVF is performed by combining the infertile couple's sperm and eggs to produce their own genetic embryos. However, unlike in standard IVF, these embryos are then transferred

Incompetent cervix

A muscular-fibrous weakening of the cervix, leading to painless cervical dilation and second-trimester or early third-trimester pregnancy loss.

Preeclampsia

A vascular disease of pregnancy characterized by hypertension, edema, and a risk of seizure.

into the uterus of the gestational carrier. This process resembles donor-egg IVF in that the process requires synchronization of two patients: the egg donor (genetic parent) and the recipient (gestational carrier). Pregnancy proceeds normally just as if the gestational carrier had become spontaneously pregnant. The major factor in determining the success rate is the age of the woman whose eggs are used. The ideal gestational carrier is a woman who has had a previous uncomplicated pregnancy and delivery.

The ideal gestational carrier is a woman who has had a previous uncomplicated pregnancy and delivery.

Complex parenting situations can arise in cases using a gestational carrier in conjunction with donor sperm, donor eggs or donor embryos. Psychological assessment of all parties is crucial and separate legal representation should be pursued by the genetic parents and the gestational carrier to ensure as smooth a transition as possible.

85. What about traditional surrogacy?

Gestational surrogacy (see Question 84 above) describes the clinical situation where the woman carrying the pregnancy is not actually genetically related to the baby that is growing in her uterus. However, traditional surrogacy refers to the situation where the egg is actually from the woman who is carrying the pregnancy. This pregnancy may have been initiated through IUI or IVF and the intent is for the woman carrying the baby to give the child to the intended parents following delivery.

The laws in many states do not permit traditional surrogacy. The rationale for this restriction is that, following delivery, the surrogate may elect to keep the baby and she would be legally allowed to do so. In general, the courts have determined that parental rights are based upon genetics, anatomy and intent. In gestational surrogacy, the carrier is not genetically related to the baby and the intent was for her to give up the baby to the genetic parents. So, even though she was carrying the baby, the courts have historically upheld the agreement. In traditional surrogacy, the surrogate contributed the egg and the womb. So, in spite of a legal agreement among all parties, the court will usually award parental rights to the surrogate because she has 2 of the 3 aspects of parental rights.

Many clinics will not participate in traditional surrogacy arrangements because of these legal issues. Individuals and couples interested in traditional surrogacy are urged to seek experienced legal advice. Lawyers practicing family law have been known to state that REs make babies but family lawyers make families.

Treatment Options: Third-Party Reproduction

PART TEN

Stress, Exercise, and Alternative Medications

What role does stress play in causing infertility?

Does being overweight have an effect on infertility or on IVF success rate?

Does smoking cause infertility?

More . . .

86. What role does stress play in causing infertility?

Not surprisingly, dealing with infertility can itself be very stressful. And stress—both physical and psychological—can significantly affect a woman's ability to conceive. A recent study examining the role of psychological stress in successful pregnancy showed a one-third decrease in pregnancy rates in those women undergoing IVF who perceived themselves to be overly stressed. Most of these women were lawyers whose stress was perceived to be job-related.

Excessive physical stress can also be detrimental to a woman's ability to conceive.

Excessive physical stress can also be detrimental to a woman's ability to conceive. Studies show that women who run more than 20 miles per week may begin to experience abnormalities in their menstrual cycle, which may in turn affect their fertility potential. Women who run marathons or compete at a very high physical level, commonly have ovulatory dysfunction and infertility.

There are many different ways to decrease the stress inherently present with infertility and its treatment—for example, decreasing work hours or changing jobs, exercise, meditation, yoga, acupuncture, getting a new hobby, or simply setting aside some time for oneself. Many patients are able to reduce their infertility-related stress by simply becoming more knowledgeable about the subject of infertility. In addition to providing physician counseling, we ask our own patients to read and become more educated about their infertility, thereby empowering them to take control of it. Excellent and reliable information is available at the American Society of Reproductive Medicine website (www.ASRM.org).

Carol comments:

Looking back on my experience, I do think that my level of stress and daily environment played a major role in my inability to conceive naturally. When I did a fresh cycle to get pregnant the second time, I had been out of the corporate environment for over a year. Not only was the quality of my embryos better, but I was able to achieve a successful pregnancy during the first fresh cycle. Obviously, it's not possible for everyone to leave their job for an extended period while attempting to get pregnant, but I do agree that anything that can be done to reduce stress is a positive contribution.

87. Can I exercise? How much is okay?

Mild to moderate exercise is beneficial to infertility patients and is highly encouraged. Healthy amounts of exercise decrease stress and clearly improve a person's sense of well-being. Studies show that women who exercise before and during their pregnancy have better obstetrical outcomes and healthier babies than women who are sedentary. For most patients, we recommend exercising 30 minutes per day, 4 or 5 times per week, but lesser amounts of exercise are still beneficial. Even 15 minutes of exercise each day can help reduce stress and improve your physical health.

We highly recommend that women begin or continue exercising during their infertility evaluation and treatments, and perhaps more so for those undergoing treatment with IVF. In our experience, these patients are better able to tolerate the stress related to infertility and IVF.

88. One of my friends tried acupuncture before her IVF cycle and it worked! Should I try acupuncture?

There is a great interest in acupuncture among fertility patients, although it is unclear whether acupuncture really improves the IVF pregnancy rates. Several studies have suggested an improvement in IVF pregnancy rates with acupuncture. In addition, acupuncture may help in decreasing the stress of infertility, which may in turn indirectly improve the likelihood for success with IVF. Decreasing stress during the infertility treatment process is always a good thing. The excellent work of Alice Domar, PhD (Domar Center for Mind/Body Health, Waltham, Massachusetts) and others has demonstrated the efficacy of the mind-body approach in relieving distress.

Along with acupuncture, there has been an increased interest in other complementary modalities including traditional Chinese herbal remedies. We remain concerned about the use of herbal medicines in patients undergoing medical treatments as many herbs can have significant side effects, including an adverse effect on the clotting cascade, resulting in an increased risk of bleeding. Our current policy is to recommend against the use of herbal medicines unless the content and potency of these supplements are clearly understood by all parties.

Kristin comments:

I looked into acupuncture during my first IVF cycle. The acupuncturist suggested that I try Reiki, a Japanese form of spiritual healing, because he preferred to treat IVF patients prior to the cycle ever starting. I can't say that Reiki got me pregnant, but it certainly helped me to relax, and that can never hurt. For women experiencing infertility, being told to "just relax" is one of the most insulting things you can hear, but if you can find a stress-reducing activity—be it yoga, massage, Reiki, acupuncture, or even meditating—it can help you to make it through the emotionally draining times.

89. Does being overweight have any effect on infertility or on IVF success rate?

Many studies show that being overweight adversely affects a woman's fertility potential and increases the likelihood for early pregnancy loss and obstetrical complications. Many obese women have irregular or absent menstrual cycles. For many of these individuals, weight reduction alone will restore their normal ovulation and menstrual cycles and enhance their fertility potential. Often, these individuals will spontaneously conceive with no medical therapy once they have reduced their weight.

Prior to performing IVF, we discuss with our patients the impact of obesity on their IVF success rates at great length. Most are very appreciative of our concern and advice, and they are generally motivated to reduce their weight so that they will have a greater chance for success with IVF and for an uncomplicated pregnancy. We recommend that obese patients—defined as those with a **body mass index (BMI)** greater than 29—reduce their weight prior to establishing pregnancy.

Sometimes it takes 2 to 6 months of weight reduction to reach the goal prior to the planned IVF treatment. Regardless of the type of infertility treatment planned, weight loss can have a dramatic effect in terms of enhancing the chance of a successful pregnancy.

Body mass index (BMI)

A mathematical calculation that uses height and weight to determine whether an individual is of normal weight, overweight, or obese.

Stress, Exercise, and Alternative Medications

161

Fad or crash diets are not recommended when a woman is trying to lose weight prior to infertility treatment, as these practices can be harmful to general health. Local community nutritionists, organizations such as Weight Watchers, personal physicians, and information available on the Internet such as the American College of Obstetricians and Gynecologists (www.ACOG.org) website can assist in establishing a plan for weight reduction.

90. Does smoking cause infertility?

Smoking significantly reduces fertility in both men and women.

Menopause

The last menstrual period that a woman ever experiences.

Smoking significantly reduces fertility in both men and women. Women who smoke are at greater risk for experiencing premature **menopause** (known as premature ovarian failure). Smoking directly affects their egg quality and egg quantity, resulting in increased rates of infertility. In IVF patients, smoking has been shown to dramatically lower the chances for a successful treatment. In addition, the chances for a spontaneous abortion are also increased in smokers compared with nonsmoking women. Smoking also directly affects sperm quality, diminishing both sperm count and sperm motility. Needless to say, quitting smoking is a good idea before pursuing fertility or fertility treatments.

91. Can I drink caffeine and alcohol during my infertility treatments?

Consumption of limited amounts of caffeine and alcohol appears to be safe when attempting to conceive. Drinking 1 to 2 cups of coffee or similar amounts of caffeinated beverages per day does not decrease a woman's chances for getting pregnant, either naturally or with any of the infertility treatments available. Although several studies suggested that drinking 1 or

2 beers or glasses of wine per day, or the equivalent, also has no adverse effect on fertility, newer information casts some doubt upon that view. Unfortunately, there are many confounding variables in this type of research; thus, we suggest that you ask your physician for his/her recommendations.

Once pregnancy occurs, limited caffeine consumption may continue without any untoward effects to the fetus. By contrast, a woman should avoid consuming even very small amounts of alcohol as soon as pregnancy occurs. Routine use of alcohol can lead to a well-recognized condition known as fetal alcohol syndrome. At this time, the consensus is that no amount of alcohol can be considered safe in pregnancy.

No amount of alcohol can be considered safe in pregnancy.

PART ELEVEN

Pregnancy Loss

How common is miscarriage?

What are the genetic causes of pregnancy loss,
and can they be treated?

Can an infection cause miscarriage?

More . . .

92. How common is miscarriage?

Human reproduction is extraordinarily inefficient. Pregnancy loss rates are remarkably high at all ages, with 10% to 15% of all clinically recognized pregnancies undergoing spontaneous abortion even in women during their peak fertility years (between 20 and 30 years old). The rate of miscarriage is age related, rising to over 50% in women older than age 40.

Many pregnancies are lost so early in development that no gestational sac is ever visualized on sonogram. This type of pregnancy loss is called a biochemical pregnancy. In most cases, once fetal cardiac activity is visualized on ultrasound, the miscarriage rate drops to less than 5%. In women older than age 40, however, the pregnancy loss rate remains 25% or greater even after visualization of cardiac activity. A pregnancy that stops developing in the absence of any bleeding is called a missed abortion. Remember that the medical term "abortion" refers to any pregnancy loss, either spontaneous or induced. Miscarriage is a lay term that is used to refer to a spontaneous abortion. Although most pregnancy losses occur during the first trimester, adverse outcomes can occur at any gestational age.

Miscarriage is a lay term that is used to refer to a spontaneous abortion.

There are many ways to manage a non-viable pregnancy. A surgical procedure called a dilation and curettage (D&C) can quickly resolve an abnormal pregnancy. In addition, the tissue from a D&C can be sent for genetic analysis to determine if the loss was genetically abnormal. Some Ob/Gyns will administer medication to induce a miscarriage using oral/vaginal drugs to initiate the miscarriage process. Finally, some physicians prefer to let nature take its course and await a spontaneous loss.

93. What can cause recurrent pregnancy loss, and can it be treated?

Given that pregnancy loss is a relatively common phenomenon, some patients might suffer several losses without any underlying predisposing factors. However, patients who suffer two or three consecutive spontaneous abortions may benefit from an evaluation to rule out any additional risk factors for poor pregnancy outcome and to determine whether any treatment might potentially reduce the risk of a recurrent loss.

Patients who suffer two or three consecutive spontaneous abortions may benefit from an evaluation.

In general, the causes of recurrent pregnancy loss can be divided into genetic, hormonal, anatomic, infectious, autoimmune, and thrombophilic categories. Approximately 40% to 50% of patients with two or three consecutive pregnancy losses will be determined to have an apparent etiology (source of the problem). In these cases, treatment would depend on the specific problem identified. In those patients without any obvious etiology of their recurrent pregnancy loss, treatment options include empiric progesterone, empiric baby aspirin, treatment with fertility medications and IUI, IVF, and IVF with preimplantation genetic diagnosis (PGD). Older patients with recurrent pregnancy loss or those with diminished ovarian reserve are probably best treated through the use of donor-egg IVF.

94. What are the genetic causes of pregnancy loss, and can they be treated?

The most common etiology of pregnancy loss is genetic. Sixty to seventy percent of first-trimester pregnancy losses are genetically not normal. The most common class of abnormality is autosomal trisomies. In such pregnancies, one extra chromosome is present in the developing pregnancy, causing it to fail. Not all trisomies

The most common class of abnormality is autosomal trisomies.

are lethal, however. For example, **trisomy** 21 (also known as Down syndrome) can result in a live birth, and children with Down syndrome are fairly well recognized by the population at large. However, most trisomy pregnancies undergo spontaneous miscarriage.

Couples who have suffered two or three consecutive losses are recommended to have their blood tested for **karyotype** analysis to ensure that they, themselves, are genetically normal. Certain chromosomal rearrangements in the parents can predispose to pregnancies possessing abnormal chromosome arrangements, leading to an increased rate of pregnancy loss or fetal abnormalities. The most common of these parental chromosomal rearrangements is a balanced translocation, in which two different chromosomes (for example, chromosomes 14 and 21) break and exchange genetic information. This rearrangement may lead to unbalanced chromosomal arrangements in the egg or the sperm, subsequently predisposing the pregnancy to miscarriage. Although patients with balanced translocations may successfully conceive and deliver healthy babies without assistance, many consider fertility treatments up to and including IVF with preimplantation genetic diagnosis (PGD) to reduce the risk of pregnancy loss. The fact that a couple has previously experienced a successful pregnancy and delivery does not preclude the possibility of a chromosomal balanced translocation.

95. Which hormonal problems can lead to miscarriage?

Several hormonal sources for pregnancy loss have been suggested, including untreated thyroid disease, diabetes, polycystic ovarian syndrome (PCOS), and luteal-phase defect.

Thyroid disease is easily diagnosed through blood tests for thyroid-stimulating hormone (TSH) and thyroid hormone itself (free T4). Fortunately, thyroid dysfunction responds promptly to treatment.

Although uncontrolled diabetes may lead to an increased risk of pregnancy loss, individuals with this degree of glucose intolerance usually have been identified prior to the pregnancy.

Women with PCOS may experience an increased risk of first-trimester pregnancy loss. It is estimated that young patients with PCOS have a 25% chance of first-trimester pregnancy loss compared with a rate of 10% to 15% in an age-matched control group. The mechanism through which PCOS may increase the chance of pregnancy loss is unknown, but limited preliminary studies suggest that the use of metformin (Glucophage) may reverse this tendency.

Women with PCOS may experience an increased risk of first-trimester pregnancy loss.

Finally, women who produce a suboptimal amount of progesterone, both in the luteal phase and in early pregnancy, are at increased risk for pregnancy loss. However, testing for such luteal-phase defects remains somewhat problematic and controversial. In our practice, we routinely supplement all patients in the first trimester of pregnancy with progesterone suppositories, obviating the need for additional diagnostic tests such as an endometrial biopsy.

96. Can fibroids or other uterine problems cause miscarriage?

Anatomical abnormalities can predispose a woman to pregnancy loss. In particular, congenital uterine abnormalities such as a uterine septum (a fibrous band separating the uterine cavity into two smaller cavities) or a unicornuate uterus (a small malformed uterus that is usually connected to a single fallopian tube) can lead to poor reproductive outcomes. Uterine malformations as a result of prenatal exposure to diethylstilbestrol (DES) can also increase a woman's risk of a poor pregnancy outcome. The presence of uterine fibroids within or abutting the endometrial cavity has been proposed as a source of pregnancy loss (see **Figure 7**); the same is true of uterine polyps. Extensive **intrauterine adhesions** from a previous dilatation and curettage (D&C) procedure may also lead to reduced reproductive success. All of

Intrauterine adhesions

Fibrous bands of tissue found within the uterine cavity.

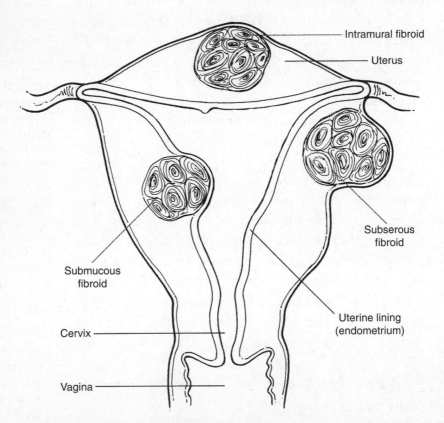

Subserous fibroids are located in the outer wall of the uterus. Intramural fibroids are found in the muscular layers of the uterine wall, and submucous fibroids are located under the uterine lining and protrude into the uterine cavity.

Figure 7   Fibroids.

Source: © 2006 American Society for Reproductive Medicine.

these abnormalities may be amenable to surgical correction, but the decision to pursue surgery requires a careful discussion with your physician.

97. Can an infection cause miscarriage?

Both bacterial and viral infectious sources for recurrent pregnancy loss have been proposed. In particular, the presence of either of two types of bacteria—ureaplasma or mycoplasma—within the cervix or uterus has been suggested as a risk factor for pregnancy loss. The scientific evidence is somewhat lacking to prove this connection, but we routinely culture our patients for ureaplasma and mycoplasma and treat both members of a sexually intimate couple when and if these bacteria are found. Women who become infected with Listeria (a type of bacterial food poisoning) after eating unpasteurized dairy products can also miscarry as a result of a uterine infection from these bacteria.

Similarly, certain viral infections can cause miscarriage if contracted during pregnancy. **Parvovirus B19** causes a mild viral illness in children known as **fifth's disease**. Children who contract this illness have a fever and bright red cheeks, lending the disease its other common name of "slapped cheek syndrome." Unfortunately, women who contract this illness during pregnancy can suffer miscarriage even in the second and third trimesters. Once infected, an individual becomes immune to this virus, so parvovirus B19 would not cause repetitive pregnancy loss. No vaccine exists for parvovirus B19.

98. Should I have autoimmune tests done if I have a history of miscarriage?

Autoimmune sources of recurrent pregnancy loss should be evaluated, especially in women with a history of

Parvovirus B19

A virus that can cause an intrauterine infection leading to fetal anemia, fetal heart failure, and miscarriage.

Fifth's disease

An infectious disease caused by parvovirus B19. It leads to bright rosy checks in children but can cause miscarriage if a woman contracts it during pregnancy.

Systemic lupus erythematosus (lupus)

A systemic autoimmune disease that causes inflammation, arthritis, rash, and other medical problems, including pregnancy loss.

Pregnancy Loss

Antiphospholipid antibodies

The general class of antibodies that are formed against various components of the cells of the body; their presence is often associated with pregnancy loss.

Anticardiolipin antibodies

Specific antibodies that are formed against various components of the cells of the body; their presence is often associated with pregnancy loss.

Women who have a history of pregnancy loss should undergo both antiphospholipid antibodies and lupus anticoagulant testing.

Thrombophilia

A disorder of the blood clotting system resulting in a tendency to form blood clots. It may also lead to a higher risk of miscarriage.

rheumatologic or autoimmune disease. Women with a preexisting autoimmune disease such as **systemic lupus erythematosus (lupus)** are clearly at risk for pregnancy loss and poor reproductive outcomes. In particular, lupus patients who have **antiphospholipid antibodies** (especially **anticardiolipin antibodies**) are at the highest risk for pregnancy loss. The presence of these antibodies in the absence of lupus also leads to an increased risk of miscarriage and poor pregnancy outcome. Treatment recommendations in such cases include daily pediatric doses of aspirin (81 mg/day), low-dose injectable blood thinners (such as heparin or Lovenox), or both.

Testing for antiphospholipid antibodies in all women who have infertility problems, even if they do not have a history of pregnancy loss, is unwarranted. In our practice, we usually restrict such testing to those patients with a history of pregnancy loss. Women who have a history of pregnancy loss should undergo both antiphospholipid antibodies and lupus anticoagulant testing.

99. What is thrombophilia, and how does it relate to miscarriage?

Over the last several years, there has been an increased interest in evaluating patients with recurrent pregnancy loss for the presence of **thrombophilia**. Thrombophilia literally means "thrombosis-loving"; a thrombosis is a blood clot. All humans exist in a balance between bleeding and blood clotting. Genetic conditions such as hemophilia leave affected individuals open to complications arising from excessive bleeding. Similarly, people who have genetic predispositions to blood clotting can be at risk for problems ranging from blood clots in the lung (pulmonary embolus) or leg (deep vein thrombosis), to an increased risk of miscarriage or poor pregnancy outcomes, including intrauterine fetal demise and intrauterine growth retardation.

Typical tests for thrombophilia include assessment of **Factor V Leiden**, **prothrombin II**, **proteins C and S**, **antithrombin III**, and the **methyltetrahydrofolate reductase (MTHFR)** enzyme. All of these, except MTHFR, are genetic enzyme deficiencies that cause the affected person to have a propensity toward blood clot formation; these conditions are often treated with pediatric aspirin and heparin (usually Lovenox).

People with an MTHFR mutation may be at higher risk for blood clot formation (and miscarriage) if they also have elevated levels of homocystine, a metabolic by-product of folic acid metabolism. People who are positive for two copies of an MTHFR enzyme mutation are best treated with vitamin supplementation consisting of folic acid, vitamin B_6, and vitamin B_{12}. Several preparations have been specifically formulated for these individuals (Foltx or Folgard). Women with thrombophilia are probably best evaluated by a hematologist to review the potential need for anticoagulation before, during, and following any pregnancy. Recent data has cast some doubt on the connection between thrombophilia and pregnancy loss, but most REs continue to test for these conditions and await definitive research.

100. Where can I go to find more information?

Appendix A lists some recommended resources for finding out more about infertility. In addition, Appendix B contains more questions and answers from the CDC's 2006 report on assisted reproductive technologies (ART).

Factor V Leiden

A genetic disorder that predisposes a woman to blood clot formation and miscarriage.

Prothrombin II

A protein involved in the blood clotting system.

Proteins C and S

Proteins involved in the blood clotting system.

Antithrombin III

A protein involved in the coagulation cascade. A deficiency in antithrombin III is associated with an increased risk of blood clotting and pregnancy loss.

Methyltetrahydrofolate reductase (MTHFR)

An enzyme involved In folic acid metabolism.

Women with thrombophilia are probably best evaluated by a hematologist to review the potential need for anticoagulation before, during, and following any pregnancy.

Pregnancy Loss

Appendix A: Patient Resources

Patient Support Groups

The American Fertility Association

The American Fertility Association is a national nonprofit organization dedicated to educating, supporting, and advocating for women and men facing decisions related to family building and reproductive health, including prevention and medical treatment of infertility, social and psychological concerns, coping mechanisms, and adoption. The AFA offers many services including publications, seminars, referrals, online educational sessions, coaching support groups, and professionally moderated message boards.

666 Fifth Avenue, Suite 278
New York, New York 10103
1-888-917-3777 (Support Line)
www.theafa.org

The Endometriosis Association

The Endometriosis Association was the first organization in the world created for those with endometriosis. As an independent self-help organization of women with endometriosis, doctors, and others interested in the disease, it is a recognized authority in its field. Its goal is to work toward finding a cure for the disease as well as providing education, support, and research.
8585 North 76th Place
Milwaukee, Wisconsin 53223
(For a free packet of information call 1-800-992-3636)
Tel: 414-355-2200
Fax: 414-355-6065
www.endometriosisassn.org

Fertile Hope

Fertile Hope is a national, nonprofit organization dedicated to providing reproductive information, support, and hope to cancer patients and survivors. Through programs of awareness, education, financial assistance, research, and support, Fertile Hope is helping cancer survivors fulfill their parenthood dreams.
Fertile Hope
Post Office Box 624
New York, New York 10014
1-888-994-HOPE
www.fertilehope.org

InterNational Council on Infertility Information Dissemination (INCIID)

The InterNational Council on Infertility Information Dissemination (INCIID—pronounced "inside") is a nonprofit organization that helps individuals and couples explore their family building options. INCIID provides current information and immediate support regarding the diagnosis, treatment, and prevention of infertility and pregnancy loss. It also offers guidance to those considering adoption or child-free lifestyles. Dr. Gordon moderates the IVF and High Tech Pregnancy Bulletin Board on the website.
Post Office Box 6836
Arlington, Virginia 22206
703-379-9178
www.inciid.org

International Premature Ovarian Failure Association (IPOFA)

The International Premature Ovarian Failure Association, Inc. (IPOFA) is a non-profit organization whose mission is to provide community, support, and information to women with Premature Ovarian Failure (POF) and their loved ones, to increase public awareness and understanding of POF, and to work with health care professionals to better understand this condition.
IPOFA
Post Office Box 23643
Alexandria, Virginia 22304
703-913-4787 (Support Line)
www.pofsupport.org

Polycystic Ovarian Syndrome Association

The Polycystic Ovarian Syndrome Association exists to provide comprehensive information, support, and advocacy for women and girls with the condition known as polycystic ovary syndrome.
Post Office Box 3403
Englewood, Colorado 80111
www.pcosupport.org

RESOLVE: The National Infertility Association

RESOLVE is a nonprofit organization mandated to promote reproductive health and to ensure equal access to all family building options for men and women experiencing infertility or other reproductive disorders. It also provides support services and physician referral and education. The mission of RESOLVE is to provide timely, compassionate support and information to people who are experiencing infertility and to increase awareness of infertility issues through public education and advocacy.
7910 Woodmont Avenue, Suite 1350
Bethesda, Maryland 20814
301-652-6611 (Main Number)
301-652-9375 (Fax)
1-888-623-0744 (Helpline)
www.resolve.org

Appendix A

Professional Organizations

American Society for Reproductive Medicine (ASRM)

American Society for Reproductive Medicine, a nonprofit organization of physicians, nurses, and other healthcare professionals, is dedicated to helping patients overcome infertility. The society accomplishes its mission through the pursuit of excellence in education and research, and through advocacy on behalf of patients, physicians, and affiliated healthcare providers.
1209 Montgomery Highway
Birmingham, Alabama 35216-2809
205-978-5000
www.asrm.org

Society for Reproductive Endocrinology and Infertility

Membership in the Society for Reproductive Endocrinology and Infertility (SREI) is limited to Board Certified Reproductive Endocrinologists. The members of the SREI are dedicated to providing excellence in reproductive health through research, education, and the care of their patients. Patients can find the reproductive endocrinologists who practice in their area by clicking on the Find Members link and can obtain additional information by viewing the pdf file for SREI physicians located at the society's website.
www.socrei.org

CDC's Assisted Reproductive Technology Page

Information is available from the CDC on reproductive health sciences. They offer statistics from infertility clinics as well as a multitude of other information pertaining to reproduction.
www.cdc.gov/ART/ART2004/index.htm

Pharmaceutical Industry

Ferring Pharmaceuticals

According to the Ferring Pharmaceuticals website:

The development of commercially available, human-derived gonadotropins has made pregnancy possible for countless women—medicines both patients and doctors can trust for consistency, purity, and reliability of results. At Ferring Pharmaceuticals, our dedication, plus more than 40 years of research and scientific expertise, has provided hope for millions of women who are struggling to conceive. Our scientists are dedicated to finding innovative solutions to help you conceive. We invite you to learn more about Ferring fertility medications at FerringFertility.com to help you fulfill your dream.

*This information is not meant to replace communications between healthcare profes-
sionals and patients. Healthcare professionals are the best source of medical information
for patients.*

Ferring provides educational materials, videos, and other free information about
their products to patients and providers.

Ferring manufactures MENOPUR®, BRAVELLE®, ENDOMETRIN® and
NOVAREL®.

Ferring Pharmaceuticals Inc.
4 Gatehall Drive, Third Floor
Parsippany, New Jersey 07054
1-888-FERRING (Customer Service Line)
www.ferringfertility.com

MERCK (formerly Organon and Schering-Plough)

Merck sponsors a website that provides more information about fertility and fertility treatment in general: Fertility Journey (*http://www.fertilityjourney.com*).
Fertility Journey is an online resource for patients. It provides information, guidance, and support as they undergo fertility treatments. Topics include: testing
and diagnosis, therapy options, and coping techniques. In addition, an online
clinic locator assists with finding a local IVF clinic for patients in
the United States.

Merck manufactures Follistim, Ganirelix, and Pregnyl. Merck
2000 Galloping Hill Road
Kenilworth, New Jersey 07033
Merck National Service Center 1-800-NSC-MERCK
http://www.fertilityjourney.com
www.merck.com
www.follistim.com

EMD Serono

According to the EMD Serono website:

*As a leader in fertility treatments, we are dedicated to providing our patients with
innovative products and continuous support for the treatment of infertility, a common
condition that affects approximately 7.3 million people in the US. We are the only
company to offer recombinant versions of three hormones used in the treatment of
infertility. These include Gonalf® (follitropin alfa for injection), Ovidrel® Prefilled
Syringe (choriogonadotropin alfa injection), and Luveris® (lutropin alfa for injection).
Rounding out EMD Serono's portfolio of fertility treatments is Cetrotide® (cetrorelix
acetate for injection) indicated for the inhibition of premature LH surges in women
undergoing controlled ovarian stimulation.*

Fertility LifeLines™ is a free, confidential, educational resource that provides customized information and support to people with fertility health concerns. A single phone call can put you in touch with customer service representatives, benefits specialists, and fertility nurses. Fertility LifeLines™ is provided by EMD Serono, a leader in fertility health.

• Visit *www.FertilityLifeLines.com*

Appendix B: SART/ CDC Annual Report

SECTION 1: OVERVIEW

Where are U.S. ART clinics located, how many ART cycles did they perform in 2006, and how many infants were born?

Although ART clinics are located throughout the United States, generally in or near major cities, the greatest number of clinics is in the eastern United States. Figure 1 shows the locations of the 426 reporting clinics. The fertility clinic section of this report, arranged in alphabetical order by state, city, and clinic name, provides specific information on each of these clinics. The number of clinics, cycles performed, live-birth deliveries, and infants born as a result

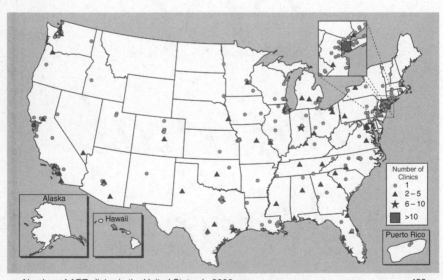

Number of ART clinics in the United States in 2006 483
Number of ART clinics that submitted data in 2006 426
Number of ART cycles reported in 2006 .... 138,198*
Number of live-birth deliveries resulting from ART cycles started in 2006 41,343
Number of infants born as a result of ART cycles carried out in 2006 54,656

Figure 1   Location of ART Clinics in the United States and Puerto Rico, 2006.

*Note: This number does not include 69 cycles in which a new treatment procedure was being evaluated (see Figure 2, page 183).

of ART all have increased steadily since CDC began collecting this information in 1995 (see Section 5, pages 235–252). Because in some cases more than one infant is born during a live-birth delivery (e.g., twins), the total number of infants born is greater than the number of live-birth deliveries. CDC estimates that ART accounts for slightly more than 1% of total U.S. births.

What types of ART cycles were used in the United States in 2006?

For 72% of ART cycles carried out in 2006, fresh nondonor eggs or embryos were used. ART cycles that used frozen nondonor embryos were the next most common type, accounting for approximately 16% of the total. In about 12% of cycles, eggs or embryos were donated by another woman. A very small number of cycles (less than 0.1% of the ART cycles carried out in 2006) involved the evaluation of a new treatment procedure. Because of the small number, cycles in which a new treatment procedure was being evaluated are not included in the total number of cycles reported in the national report or in the individual fertility clinic tables. Thus, data presented

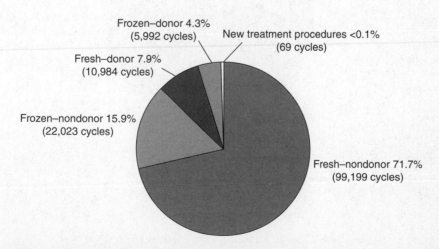

Figure 2   Types of ART Cycles—United States,* 2006.

*Total does not equal 100% due to rounding.

in subsequent figures in this report and in the individual fertility clinic tables are based on 138,198 ART cycles.

How old were the women who used ART in the United States in 2006?

The average age of women using ART services in 2006 was 36. The largest group of women using ART services were women younger than 35, representing 39% of all ART cycles carried out in 2006. Twenty-three percent of ART cycles were carried out among women aged 35–37, 19% among women aged 38–40, 10% among women aged 41–42, and 10% among women older than 42 (see Figure 3).

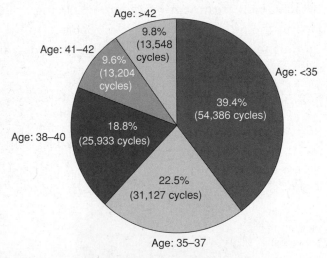

Figure 3   ART Use by Age Group—United States,* 2006.

*Total does not equal 100% due to rounding.

How did the types of ART cycles used in the United States in 2006 differ among women of different ages?

Figure 4 shows that, in 2006, the type of ART cycles varied by the woman's age. The vast majority (96%) of women younger than 35 used their own eggs, whereas only 4% used donor eggs. In contrast, 21% of women aged 41 to 42 and more than half (55%) of women older than 42 used donor eggs. Across all age groups, more ART cycles using fresh eggs or embryos were performed than cycles using frozen embryos.

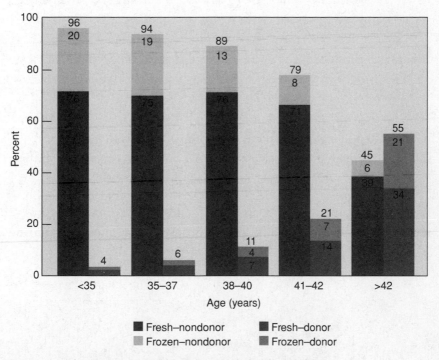

Figure 4   Types of ART Cycles by Age Group—United States, 2006.

SECTION 2: ART CYCLES USING FRESH NONDONOR EGGS OR EMBRYOS

What are the steps for an ART cycle using fresh nondonor eggs or embryos?

Figure 5 presents the steps for an ART cycle using fresh nondonor eggs or embryos and shows how ART users in 2006 progressed through these stages toward pregnancy and live birth.

An ART **cycle is started** when a woman begins taking medication to stimulate the ovaries to develop eggs or, if no drugs are given, when the woman begins having her ovaries monitored (using ultra-sound or blood tests) for natural egg production.

If eggs are produced, the cycle then progresses to **egg retrieval**, a surgical procedure in which eggs are collected from a woman's ovaries.

Once retrieved, eggs are combined with sperm in the laboratory. If fertilization is successful, one or more of the resulting embryos are selected for **transfer**, most often into a woman's uterus through the cervix (IVF), but sometimes into the fallopian tubes.

If one or more of the transferred embryos implant within the woman's uterus, the cycle then may progress to clinical **pregnancy**.

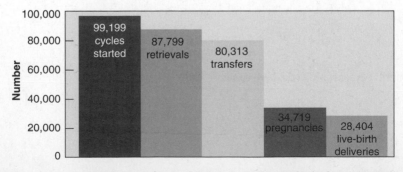

Figure 5   Outcome of ART Cycles Using Fresh Nondonor Eggs or Embryos, by Stage, 2006.

Finally, the pregnancy may progress to a **live birth**, the delivery of one or more live-born infants. (The birth of twins, triplets, or more is counted as one live birth.)

A cycle may be discontinued at any step for specific medical reasons (e.g., no eggs are produced, the embryo transfer was not successful) or by patient choice.

Why are some ART cycles discontinued?

In 2006, 11,400 ART cycles (about 11%) were discontinued before the egg retrieval step (see Figure 5, page 186). Figure 6 shows reasons that the cycles were stopped. For approximately 84% of these cycles, there was no or inadequate egg production. Other reasons included too high a response to ovarian stimulation medications (i.e., potential for ovarian hyperstimulation syndrome), concurrent medical illness, or a patient's personal reasons.

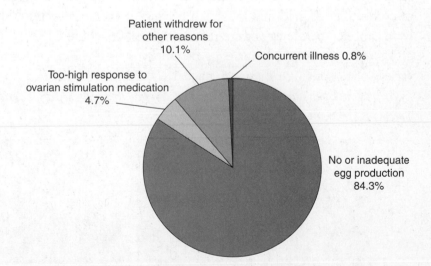

Figure 6   Reasons ART Cycles Using Fresh Nondonor Eggs or Embryos Were Discontinued,*† 2006.

*Based on 11,400 ART cycles.
†Total does not equal 100% due to rounding.

Appendix B

How is the success of ART measured?

Figure 7 shows ART success rates using six different measures, each providing slightly different information about this complex process. The vast majority of success rates have increased slightly each year since CDC began monitoring them in 1995 (see Section 5, pages 235–252).

- **Percentage of ART cycles started that produced a pregnancy:** This is higher than the percentage of cycles that resulted in a live birth because some pregnancies end in miscarriage, induced abortion, or stillbirth (see Figure 9, page 190).
- **Percentage of ART cycles started that resulted in a live birth (a delivery of one or more live-born infants):** This is the one many people are most interested in because it represents the average chance of having a live-born infant by using ART. *This is referred to as the basic live birth rate in the Fertility Clinic Success Rate and Certification Act of 1992.*
- **Percentage of ART cycles in which eggs were retrieved that resulted in a live birth:** This is generally higher than the percentage of cycles that resulted in a live birth because it excludes cycles that were canceled before eggs were retrieved. In 2006, about 11% of all cycles using fresh nondonor eggs or embryos were canceled for a variety of reasons (see Figure 6, page 187). *This is referred to as the live birth rate per successful oocyte (egg) retrieval in the Fertility Clinic Success Rate and Certification Act of 1992.*

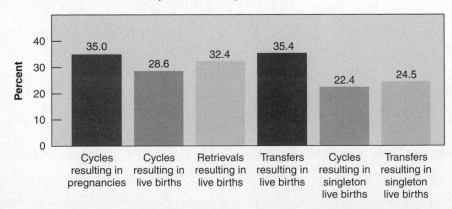

Figure 7   Success Rates for ART Cycles Using Fresh Nondonor Eggs or Embryos, by Different Measures, 2006.

- **Percentage of ART cycles in which an embryo or egg and sperm transfer occurred that resulted in a live birth:** This is the highest of these six measures of ART success.
- **Percentage of ART cycles started that resulted in a singleton live birth:** Overall, singleton live births have a much lower risk than multiple-infant births for adverse infant health outcomes, including prematurity, low birth weight, disability, and death.
- **Percentage of ART cycles in which an embryo or egg and sperm transfer occurred that resulted in a singleton live birth:** This is higher than the percentage of ART cycles started that resulted in a singleton live birth because not all ART cycles proceed to embryo transfer.

What percentage of ART cycles results in a pregnancy?

Figure 8 shows the results of ART cycles in 2006 that used fresh nondonor eggs or embryos. Most of these cycles (64%) did not produce a pregnancy; a very small proportion (0.7%) resulted in an

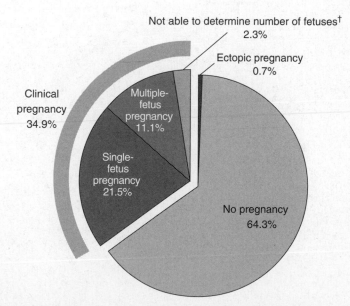

Figure 8   Results of ART Cycles Using Fresh Nondonor Eggs or Embryos,* 2006.

*Total does not equal 100% due to rounding.

†Number of fetuses not known because the pregnancy ended in an early miscarriage.

ectopic pregnancy (the embryo implanted outside the uterus), and 35% resulted in clinical pregnancy. Clinical pregnancies can be further subdivided as follows:

- 21.5% resulted in a single-fetus pregnancy.
- 11.1% resulted in a multiple-fetus pregnancy.
- 2.3% ended in miscarriage before the number of fetuses could be accurately determined.

What percentage of pregnancies results in a live birth?

Figure 9 shows the outcomes of pregnancies resulting from ART cycles in 2006 (see Figure 8, page 189). Approximately 82% of the pregnancies resulted in a live birth (57% in a singleton birth and 25% in a multiple-infant birth). About 18% of pregnancies resulted in an adverse outcome (miscarriage, stillbirth, induced abortion, or maternal death). For 0.6% of pregnancies, the outcome was unknown.

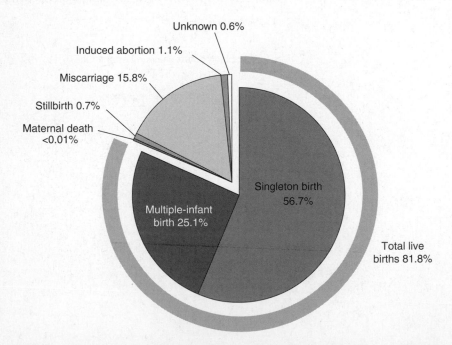

Figure 9   Outcomes of Pregnancies Resulting from ART Cycles Using Fresh Nondonor Eggs or Embryos,* 2006.

*Total does not equal 100% due to rounding.

Although the birth of more than one infant is counted as one live birth, multiple-infant births are presented here as a separate category because they often are associated with problems for both mothers and infants. Infant deaths and birth defects are not included as adverse outcomes because the available information for these outcomes is incomplete.

Using ART, what is the risk of having a multiple-fetus pregnancy or multiple-infant live birth?

Multiple-infant births are associated with greater problems for both mothers and infants, including higher rates of caesarean section, prematurity, low birth weight, and infant disability or death.

Part A of Figure 10 shows that among the 34,719 pregnancies that resulted from ART cycles using fresh nondonor eggs or embryos, 62% were singleton pregnancies, 28% were twins, and about 4% were triplets or more. Seven percent of pregnancies ended in miscarriage in which the number of fetuses could not be accurately determined.

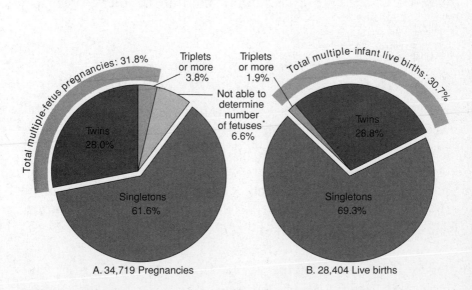

Figure 10   Risks of Having Multiple-Fetus Pregnancy and Multiple-Infant Live Birth from ART Cycles Using Fresh Nondonor Eggs or Embryos, 2006.

*Number of fetuses not known because the pregnancy ended in an early miscarriage.

Therefore, the percentage of pregnancies with more than one fetus might have been higher than what was reported (about 32%).

In 2006, 6,117 pregnancies resulting from ART cycles ended in either miscarriage, stillbirth, induced abortion, or maternal death, and 198 pregnancy outcomes were not reported. The remaining 28,404 pregnancies resulted in live births. Part B of Figure 10 shows that approximately 31% of these live births produced more than one infant (29% twins and approximately 2% triplets or more). This compares with a multiple-infant birth rate of slightly more than 3% in the general U.S. population.

Although the total rates for multiples were similar between pregnancies and live births, there were more triplet-or-more pregnancies than births. Triplet-or-more pregnancies may be reduced to twins or singletons by the time of birth. This can happen naturally (e.g., fetal death), or a woman and her doctor may decide to reduce the number of fetuses using a procedure called multifetal pregnancy reduction. CDC does not collect information on multifetal pregnancy reductions.

Using ART, what is the risk for preterm birth?

Preterm birth occurs when a woman gives birth before 37 full weeks of pregnancy. Infants born preterm are at greater risk for death in the first few days of life, as well as other adverse health outcomes including mental retardation, visual and hearing impairments, learning disabilities, and behavioral and emotional problems throughout life. Preterm births also cause substantial emotional and economic burdens for families.

Figure 11 shows percentages of preterm births resulting from ART cycles that used fresh nondonor eggs or embryos, by the number of infants born. For singletons, it shows separately the preterm percentage for pregnancies that started with one fetus (single-fetus pregnancies) or more than one (multiple-fetus pregnancies).

Appendix B

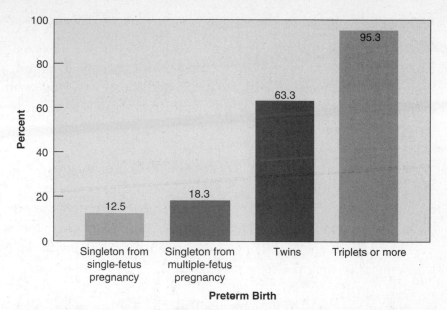

Figure 11 **Percentages of Preterm Births from ART Cycles Using Fresh Nondonor Eggs or Embryos, by Number of Infants Born, 2006.**

Among singletons, the percentage of preterm births was higher for those from multiple-fetus pregnancies (18%) than those from single-fetus pregnancies (12%). In the general U.S. population, where singletons are almost always the result of a single-fetus pregnancy, 13% were born preterm in 2005 (most recent available data).

Among ART births, 63% of twins and 95% of triplets or more were born preterm. A comparison of preterm births between ART twins and triplets or more and similar births in the general population is not meaningful because the vast majority of multiple-infant births in the United States are due to infertility treatments (both ART and non-ART).

These data indicate that the risk for preterm birth is higher among infants conceived through ART than for infants in the general population. This increase in risk is, in large part, due to the higher rate of multiple-infant pregnancies resulting from ART cycles.

Using ART, what is the risk of having low-birth-weight infants?

Low-birth-weight infants (less than 2,500 grams, or 5 pounds, 9 ounces) are at increased risk for death and short- and long-term disabilities such as cerebral palsy, mental retardation, and limitations in motor and cognitive skills.

Figure 12 presents percentages of low-birth-weight infants resulting from ART cycles that used fresh nondonor eggs or embryos, by number of infants born. For singletons, it shows separately the percentages of low birth weight among infants born from pregnancies that started with one fetus (single-fetus pregnancies) and with more than one fetus (multiple-fetus pregnancies).

Among singletons born through ART, the percentage of low-birth-weight infants was higher for those from multiple-fetus pregnancies (17%) than those from single-fetus pregnancies (8%). In the general U.S. population, where singletons are almost always the result of a single-fetus pregnancy, 8% of infants born in 2005 (most recent available data) had low birth weights.

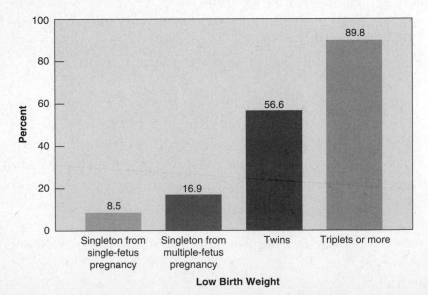

Figure 12   Percentages of Low-Birth-Weight Infants from ART Cycles Using Fresh Nondonor Eggs or Embryos, by Number of Infants Born, 2006.

Approximately 57% of twins and 90% of triplets or more had low birth weights. Comparing percentages of low birth weight between ART twins and triplets or more and the general population is not meaningful because the vast majority of multiple births in the United States are due to infertility treatments (both ART and non-ART).

These data indicate that the risk for low birth weight is higher for infants conceived through ART than for infants in the general population. The increase in risk is due, in large part, to the higher percentage of multiple-infant pregnancies resulting from ART cycles.

What are the ages of women who use ART?

Figure 13 presents ART cycles using fresh nondonor eggs or embryos according to the age of the woman who had the procedure. About 12% of these cycles were among women younger than age 30, 67% were among women aged 30–39, and approximately 21% were among women aged 40 and older.

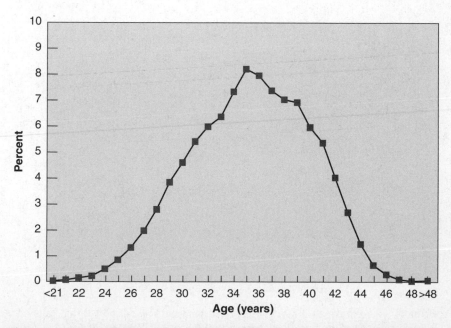

Figure 13 Age Distribution of Women Who Had ART Cycles Using Fresh Nondonor Eggs or Embryos, 2006.

Do ART success rates differ among women of different ages?

A woman's age is the most important factor affecting the chances of a live birth when her own eggs are used. Figure 14 shows the percentages of pregnancies, live births, and singleton live births for women of different ages who had ART procedures using fresh nondonor eggs or embryos in 2006. The percentages of ART cycles resulting in live births and singleton live births are different because of the high percentage of multiple-infant deliveries counted among the total live births. The percentage of multiple-infant births is particularly high among women younger than 35 (see Figure 34, page 217). Among women in their 20s, the percentages of ART cycles resulting in pregnancies, live births, and singleton live births were relatively stable; however, success rates declined steadily from the mid-30s onward. For additional detail on success rates among women aged 40 or older, see Figure 15 on page 197.

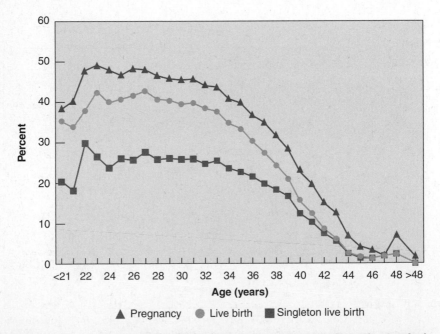

Figure 14 Percentages of ART Cycles Using Fresh Nondonor Eggs or Embryos That Resulted in Pregnancies, Live Births, and Singleton Live Births, by Age of Woman,* 2006.

*For consistency, all percentages are based on cycles started.

How do ART success rates differ for women who are 40 or older?

Success rates decline with each year of age and are particularly low for women 40 or older. Figure 15 shows the percentages of pregnancies, live births, and singleton live births in 2006 for women 40 or older who used fresh nondonor eggs or embryos. The average chance for pregnancy was 23% for women age 40; the percentage of ART cycles resulting in live births for this age was about 15%, and the percentage of ART cycles resulting in singleton live births was about 12%. All percentages dropped steadily with each 1-year increase in age. For women older than 44, the percentages of live births and singleton live births were both a little more than 1%. Women 40 or older generally have much higher success rates using donor eggs (see Figure 45, page 230).

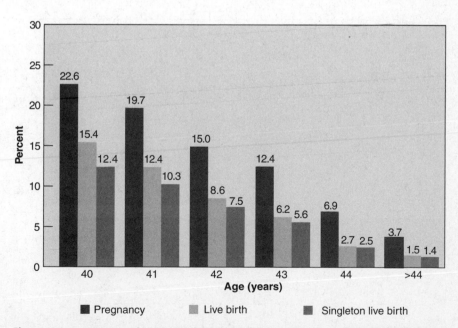

Figure 15   Percentages of ART Cycles Using Fresh Nondonor Eggs or Embryos That Resulted in Pregnancies, Live Births, and Singleton Live Births Among Women Aged 40 or Older,* 2006.

*For consistency, all percentages are based on cycles started.

How does the risk for miscarriage differ among women of different ages?

A woman's age not only affects the chance for pregnancy when her own eggs are used, but also affects her risk for miscarriage. Figure 16 shows the percentages of ART cycles started in 2006 that resulted in miscarriage for women of different ages. The percentages of ART cycles that resulted in miscarriage were below 14% among women younger than 35. The percentages of ART cycles that resulted in miscarriages began to increase among women in their mid- to late 30s and continued to increase with age, reaching 28% at age 40 and 56% among women older than 43.

The risk for miscarriage observed among women undergoing ART procedures using fresh nondonor eggs or embryos appears to be similar to that reported in various studies of other pregnant women in the United States.

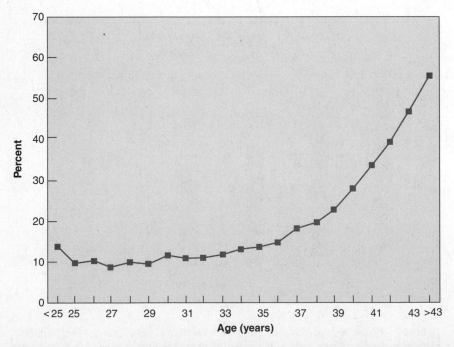

Figure 16 Percentages of ART Cycles Using Fresh Nondonor Eggs or Embryos That Resulted in Miscarriage, by Age of Woman, 2006.

What is the risk for pregnancy loss at different times during pregnancy among women of different ages?

A woman's risk for pregnancy loss (loss of an entire pregnancy, or all fetuses in a multiple-fetus pregnancy) is affected by the duration of her pregnancy and her age. Figure 17 shows that between 13% and 52% of clinically-detected pregnancies (clinical detection through ultrasound performed between 4 and 6 weeks after the day of embryo transfer) are lost at some later point during the pregnancy, depending on the woman's age. Among women younger than 35, 13% of pregnancies were lost and 87% continued through week 24. In contrast, among women older than 42, 52% of pregnancies were lost and only 48% continued through week 24. In all age groups, most pregnancy losses occurred before week 14 (i.e., during the first trimester). The risk of pregnancy loss after 24 weeks was less than 1% for all age groups because most pregnancies that progress beyond week 24 lead to live births.

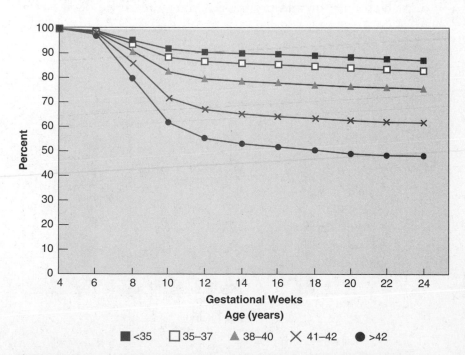

Figure 17   Percentages of Pregnancies That Continued Past a Given Gestational Week Among Women Who Had ART Cycles Using Fresh Nondonor Eggs or Embryos, by Age of Woman, 2006.

Appendix B

How does a woman's age affect her chances of progressing through the various stages of ART?

In 2006, a total of 99,199 cycles using fresh nondonor eggs or embryos were started:

- 41,369 in women younger than 35
- 23,376 in women 35–37
- 19,775 in women 38–40
- 9,346 in women 41–42
- 5,333 in women older than 42

Figure 18 shows that a woman's chance of progressing from the beginning of ART to pregnancy and live birth (using her own eggs) decreases at every stage of ART as her age increases.

- As women get older, the likelihood of a successful response to ovarian stimulation and progression to **egg retrieval** decreases.
- As women get older, cycles that have progressed to egg retrieval are slightly less likely to reach **transfer**.

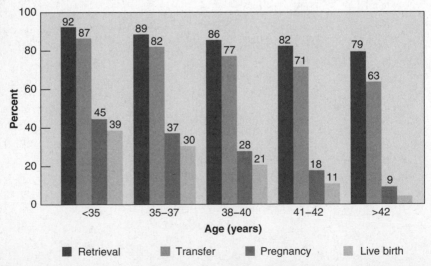

Figure 18   Outcomes of ART Cycles Using Fresh Nondonor Eggs or Embryos, by Stage and Age Group, 2006.

- The percentage of cycles that progress from transfer to **pregnancy** also decreases as women get older.
- As women get older, cycles that have progressed to pregnancy are less likely to result in a **live birth** because the risk for miscarriage is greater (see Figure 16, page 198).

Overall, 39% of cycles started in 2006 among women younger than 35 resulted in live births. This percentage decreased to 30% among women 35–37 years of age, 21% among women 38–40, 11% among women 41–42, and 4% among women older than 42. As noted in Figures 14 and 15 (see pages 196 and 197), the proportion of cycles that resulted in singleton live births is even lower for each age group.

What are the causes of infertility among couples who use ART?

Figure 19 shows the infertility diagnoses reported among couples who had an ART procedure using fresh nondonor eggs or embryos in 2006. Diagnoses range from one infertility factor in one partner to multiple factors in either one or both partners. However, diagnostic

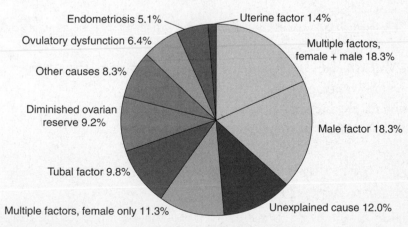

Endometriosis 5.1%
Uterine factor 1.4%
Ovulatory dysfunction 6.4%
Multiple factors, female + male 18.3%
Other causes 8.3%
Diminished ovarian reserve 9.2%
Male factor 18.3%
Tubal factor 9.8%
Multiple factors, female only 11.3%
Unexplained cause 12.0%

Figure 19 Diagnoses Among Couples Who Had ART Cycles Using Fresh Nondonor Eggs or Embryos,* 2006.

*Total does not equal 100% due to rounding.

procedures may vary from one clinic to another, so the categorization may also vary.

- **Tubal factor** means that the woman's fallopian tubes are blocked or damaged, making it difficult for the egg to be fertilized or for an embryo to travel to the uterus.
- **Ovulatory dysfunction** means that the ovaries are not producing eggs normally. Such dysfunctions include polycystic ovary syndrome and multiple ovarian cysts.
- **Diminished ovarian reserve** means that the ability of the ovary to produce eggs is reduced. Reasons include congenital, medical, or surgical causes or advanced age.
- **Endometriosis** involves the presence of tissue similar to the uterine lining in abnormal locations. This condition can affect both fertilization of the egg and embryo implantation.
- **Uterine factor** means a structural or functional disorder of the uterus that results in reduced fertility.
- **Male factor** refers to a low sperm count or problems with sperm function that make it difficult for a sperm to fertilize an egg under normal conditions.
- **Other causes** of infertility include immunological problems, chromosomal abnormalities, cancer chemotherapy, and serious illnesses.
- **Unexplained cause** means that no cause of infertility was found in either the woman or the man.
- **Multiple factors, female only,** means that more than one female cause was diagnosed.
- **Multiple factors, female and male,** means that one or more female causes and male factor infertility were diagnosed.

Does the cause of infertility affect the chances of success using ART?

Figure 20 shows the percentage of ART cycles that resulted in live births according to the causes of infertility. (See Figure 19, page 201, for an explanation of the diagnoses.) Although the national average success rate was about 29% (see Figure 7, page 188), success rates varied somewhat depending on the couple's diagnosis; however, the definitions of these diagnoses may vary from clinic to clinic. In general, couples diagnosed with tubal factor, ovulatory dysfunction, endometriosis, male factor, or unexplained infertility had success rates above the national average. The lowest success rate was observed for those with diminished ovarian reserve. Additionally, couples with uterine factor, "other" causes, or multiple infertility factors had below-average success rates. Please note, however, that a review of select clinical records revealed that reporting of infertility causes may be incomplete. Therefore, differences in success rates by causes of infertility should be interpreted with caution.

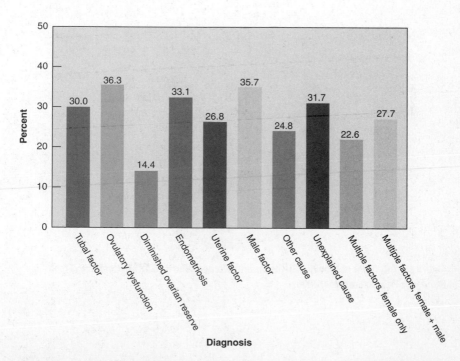

Figure 20   Percentages of ART Cycles Using Fresh Nondonor Eggs or Embryos That Resulted in Live Births, by Diagnosis, 2006.

How many women who use ART have previously given birth?

Figure 21 shows the number of previous births among women who had an ART procedure using fresh nondonor eggs or embryos in 2006. Most of these women (71%) had no previous births, although they may have had a pregnancy that resulted in a miscarriage or an induced abortion. Twenty-one percent of women using ART in 2006 reported one previous birth, and about 8% reported two or more previous births. However, we do not have information about how many of these were ART births and how many were not. These data nonetheless point out that women who have previously had children can still face infertility problems.

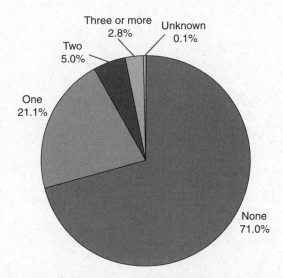

Figure 21   Number of Previous Births Among Women Who Had ART Cycles Using Fresh Nondonor Eggs or Embryos, 2006.

Do women who have previously given birth have higher ART success rates?

Figure 22 shows the relationship between the success of an ART cycle and the woman's history of previous births. Previous live-born infants were conceived naturally in some cases and through ART in others. In all age groups, women who had a previous live birth were more likely to have a successful ART procedure.

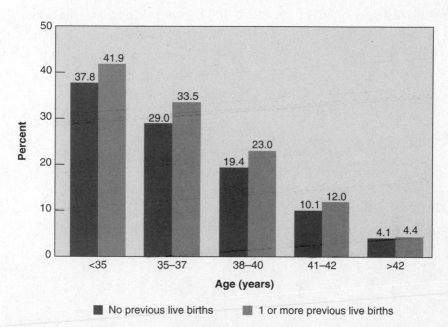

Figure 22   Percentages of ART Cycles Using Fresh Nondonor Eggs or Embryos That Resulted in Live Births, by Woman's Age and Number of Previous Live Births, 2006.

Is there a difference in ART success rates between women with previous miscarriages and women who have never been pregnant?

In 2006, 70,428 ART cycles were performed among women who had not previously given birth. However, about 27% of those cycles were reported by women with one or more previous pregnancies that had ended in miscarriage—we do not have information on whether these pregnancies ending in miscarriage were the result of ART or were conceived naturally. Figure 23 shows the relationship between the success of an ART cycle and the history of previous miscarriage. In all age groups, women who had a previous miscarriage were as likely to have a live birth as women who had never been pregnant. Thus, a history of unsuccessful pregnancy does not appear to be associated with lower chances for success during ART.

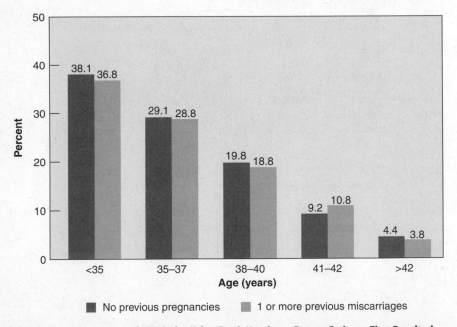

Figure 23   Percentages of ART Cycles Using Fresh Nondonor Eggs or Embryos That Resulted in Live Births, by Woman's Age and History of Miscarriage, Among Women with No Previous Births,* 2006.

*Women reporting only previous ectopic pregnancies or pregnancies that ended in induced abortion were not included in the above statistics.

How many current ART users have undergone previous ART cycles?

Figure 24 presents ART cycles that used fresh nondonor eggs or embryos in 2006 according to whether previous ART cycles had been performed. For about 43%, one or more previous cycles were reported. (This percentage includes previous cycles using either fresh or frozen embryos.) This finding illustrates that it is not uncommon for a couple to undergo multiple ART cycles. We do not have information on when previous cycles were performed, nor do we have information on the outcomes of those previous cycles.

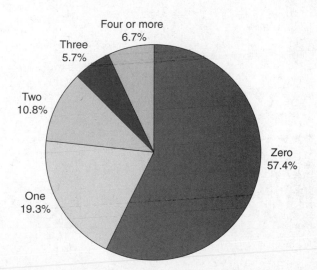

Figure 24   Number of Previous ART Cycles Among Women Undergoing ART with Fresh Nondonor Eggs or Embryos,* 2006.

*Total does not equal 100% due to rounding.

Appendix B

Are success rates different for women using ART for the first time and women who previously used ART but did not give birth?

Figure 25 shows the relationship between the success of ART cycles performed in 2006 using fresh nondonor eggs or embryos and a history of previous ART cycles among women with no previous births. In all age groups up to age 42, success rates were lower for women who had previously undergone an unsuccessful ART cycle.

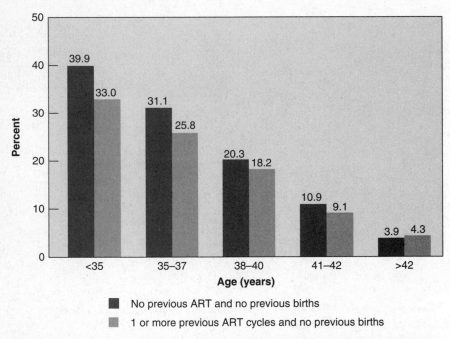

Figure 25   Percentages of ART Cycles Using Fresh Nondonor Eggs or Embryos That Resulted in Live Births, by Woman's Age and History of Previous ART Cycles, Among Women with No Previous Births, 2006.

What are the success rates for women who have had both *previous ART and previous births?*

Figure 26 shows the relationship between the success of ART cycles performed in 2006 using fresh nondonor eggs or embryos and a history of both previous ART cycles and previous births. We do not have information on whether the previous births were the result of ART or were conceived naturally. However, among women with previous births, success rates among women who did not undergo a previous ART procedure were comparable to success rates among women who had undergone previous ART cycles.

Taken together, Figures 25 (see page 208) and 26 show that having undergone previous ART cycles may be related to the success of the current ART cycle. However, it is important to consider the outcomes of previous cycles and whether the woman has given birth in the past.

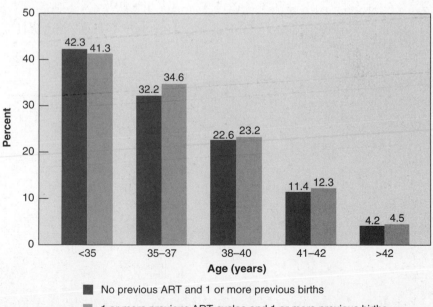

Figure 26   Percentages of ART Cycles Using Fresh Nondonor Eggs or Embryos That Resulted in Live Births, by Woman's Age and History of Previous ART Cycles, Among Women with One or More Previous Births, 2006.

What were the specific types of ART performed among women who used fresh nondonor eggs or embryos in 2006?

For about 38% of ART procedures that used fresh nondonor eggs or embryos in 2006, standard IVF (in vitro fertilization) techniques were used: eggs and sperm were combined in the laboratory, the resulting embryos were cultured for 2 or more days, and one or more embryos were then transferred into the woman's uterus through the cervix.

For most of the remaining ART procedures (62%), fertilization was accomplished using intracytoplasmic sperm injection (ICSI). This technique involves injecting a single sperm directly into an egg; the embryos are then cultured and transferred as in standard IVF.

For a small proportion of ART procedures, unfertilized eggs and sperm (gametes) or early embryos (zygotes) were transferred into the woman's fallopian tubes. These procedures are known as gamete and zygote intrafallopian transfer (GIFT and ZIFT). Some women with tubal infertility are not suitable candidates for GIFT and ZIFT.

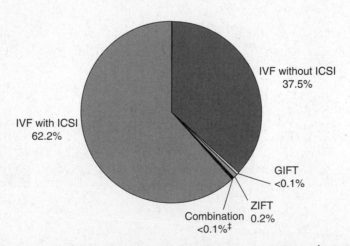

Figure 27   Types of ART Procedures Using Fresh Nondonor Eggs or Embryos,*† 2006.

*Cycles that were canceled before egg retrieval were classified as IVF, GIFT, or ZIFT based on the intended ART method.
†Total does not equal 100% due to rounding.
‡Combination of IVF with or without ICSI and either GIFT or ZIFT.

GIFT and ZIFT are more invasive procedures than IVF because they involve inserting a laparoscope into a woman's abdomen to transfer the embryos or gametes into the fallopian tubes. In contrast, IVF involves transferring embryos or gametes into a woman's uterus through the cervix without surgery.

What are the success rates for different types of ART procedures?

Figure 28 shows the percentage of egg retrievals that resulted in a live birth for each type of ART procedure started in 2006. Success rates for the two predominant types of ART, IVF without ICSI and IVF with ICSI, were similar. The success rates for cycles that used GIFT, ZIFT, or a combination of IVF were much lower than for cycles that used other ART procedures. See Figures 29–31 (pages 212–214) and Figures 50–55 (pages 236–243) for further details on IVF procedures that used ICSI.

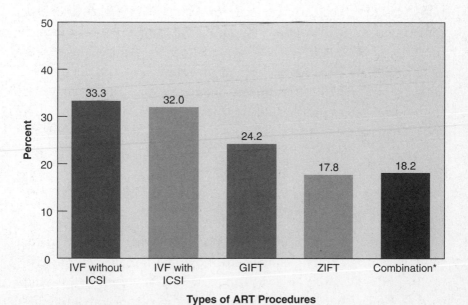

Figure 28   Percentages of Egg Retrievals That Resulted in Live Births, by Type of ART Procedure, 2006.

*Combination of IVF with or without ICSI and either GIFT or ZIFT.

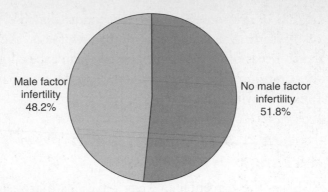

Figure 29   Use of ICSI* in Fresh– Nondonor Cycles Among Couples With and Without Diagnoses of Male Factor Infertility,[†] 2006.

*Intracytoplasmic sperm injection.
[†]Based on 61,722 cycles that used IVF with ICSI.

Is ICSI used only for couples diagnosed with male factor infertility?

ICSI was developed to overcome problems with fertilization that sometimes occur in couples diagnosed with male factor infertility. In 2006, 61,722 ICSI cycles were performed. Approximately half of the ICSI cycles were performed for couples with a diagnosis of male factor infertility. However, diagnostic procedures may vary from one clinic to another, so the categorization of causes of infertility may also vary.

What are the success rates for couples with male factor infertility when ICSI is used?

ICSI was developed to overcome problems with fertilization that sometimes occur among couples diagnosed with male factor infertility. In 2006, 82% of couples diagnosed with male factor infertility used IVF with ICSI. Figure 30 presents the success rates for these ICSI procedures among couples diagnosed with male factor infertility. For comparison, these rates are presented alongside the success rates for ART cycles that used standard IVF without ICSI.

This standard IVF comparison group includes couples with all diagnoses except male factor. Because ICSI can be performed only when at least one egg has been retrieved, the percentages of egg retrievals that resulted in live births are presented.

In every age group, success rates for the IVF with ICSI group were similar to the success rates for the groups that used standard IVF without ICSI. These results show that when ICSI was used for couples diagnosed with male factor infertility, their success rates were close to those achieved by couples who were not diagnosed with male factor infertility. Please note, however, that review of select clinical records revealed that reporting of infertility causes may be incomplete. Therefore, differences in success rates by causes of infertility should be interpreted with caution.

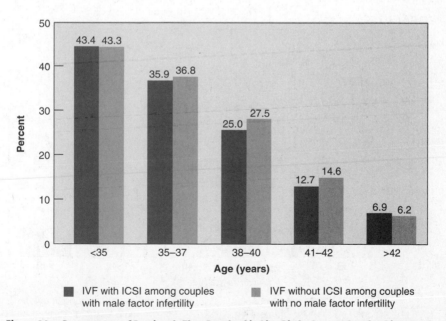

Figure 30   Percentages of Retrievals That Resulted in Live Births Among Couples Diagnosed with Male Factor Infertility Who Used IVF with ICSI,* Compared with Couples Not Diagnosed with Male Factor Infertility Who Used IVF Without ICSI, by Woman's Age,[†] 2006.

*Intracytoplasmic sperm injection.
[†]Cycles using donor sperm and cycles using GIFT or ZIFT are excluded.

What are the success rates for couples without a diagnosis of male factor infertility when ICSI is used?

As shown in Figure 29 (page 212), a large number of ICSI procedures are now performed even when couples are not diagnosed with male factor infertility. Figure 31 presents percentages of egg retrievals that resulted in live births for those cycles compared with ART cycles among couples who used IVF without ICSI. For every age group, the ICSI procedures were less successful. Please note, however, that review of select clinical records revealed that reporting of infertility causes may be incomplete. Therefore, differences in success rates by causes of infertility should be interpreted with caution. Additionally, information was not available to completely determine whether this finding was directly related to the ICSI procedure or whether the patients who used ICSI were somehow different from those who use IVF alone. However, separate evaluation of various groups of

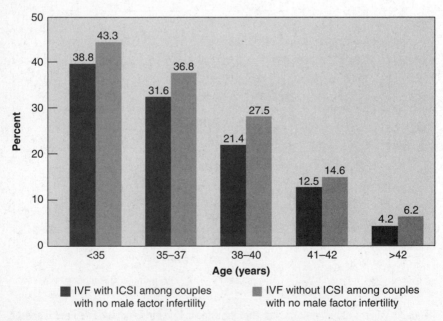

Figure 31 Percentages of Retrievals That Resulted in Live Births Among Couples Not Diagnosed with Male Factor Infertility, by Use of ICSI* and Woman's Age,[†] 2006.

*Intracytoplasmic sperm injection.
[†]Cycles using donor sperm and cycles using GIFT or ZIFT are excluded.

patients with an indication of being difficult to treat revealed a pattern of results consistent with those presented below. These difficult-to-treat groups included couples with previous failed ART cycles, couples diagnosed with diminished ovarian reserve, and couples with a low number of eggs retrieved (fewer than five). Within each of these groups, ART cycles that used IVF with ICSI had lower success rates compared with cycles that used IVF without ICSI.

How many embryos are transferred in an ART procedure?

Figure 32 shows that approximately 43% of ART cycles that used fresh nondonor eggs or embryos and progressed to the embryo transfer stage in 2006 involved the transfer of three or more embryos, about 16% of cycles involved the transfer of four or more, and approximately 5% of cycles involved the transfer of five or more embryos.

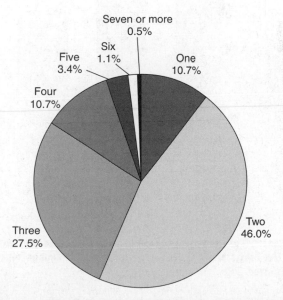

Figure 32   Number of Embryos Transferred During ART Cycles Using Fresh Nondonor Eggs or Embryos,* 2006.

*Total does not equal 100% due to rounding.

In general, is an ART cycle more likely to be successful if more embryos are transferred?

Figure 33 shows the relationship between the number of embryos transferred during an ART procedure in 2006 and the number of infants born alive as a result of that procedure. The success rate increased when two or more embryos were transferred; however, transferring multiple embryos also poses a risk of having a multiple-infant birth. Multiple-infant births cause concern because of the additional health risks they create for both mothers and infants. Also, pregnancies with multiple fetuses are potentially subject to multifetal reduction. Multifetal reduction can happen naturally (e.g., fetal death), or a woman or couple may decide to reduce the number of fetuses using a procedure called multifetal pregnancy reduction.

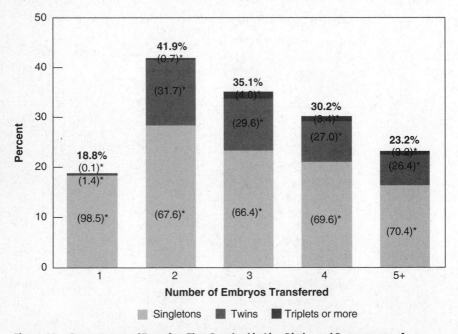

Figure 33   Percentages of Transfers That Resulted in Live Births and Percentages of Multiple-Infant Live Births for ART Cycles Using Fresh Nondonor Eggs or Embryos, by Number of Embryos Transferred, 2006.

*Percentages of live births that were singletons, twins, and triplets or more are in parentheses.
Note: In rare cases a single embryo may divide and thus produce twins. For this reason, a small percentage of twins resulted from a single embryo transfer, and a small percentage of triplets resulted when two embryos were transferred.

Information on multifetal pregnancy reductions is incomplete and therefore is not provided here.

The relationships between number of embryos transferred, success rates, and multiple-infant births are complicated by several factors, such as the woman's age and embryo quality. See Figure 34 (page 217) for more details on women most at risk for multiple births.

Are success rates affected by the number of embryos transferred for women who have more embryos available than they choose to transfer?

Although, in general, transferring more than one embryo tends to improve the chance for a successful ART procedure (see Figure 33, page 216), other factors are also important. Previous research suggests that the number of embryos fertilized and thus available for ART

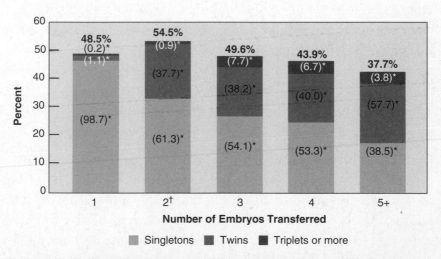

Figure 34   Percentages of Transfers That Resulted in Live Births and Percentages of Multiple-Infant Live Births for ART Cycles in Women Who Were Younger Than 35, Used Fresh Nondonor Eggs or Embryos, and Set Aside Extra Embryos for Future Use, by Number of Embryos Transferred, 2006.

*Percentages of live births that were singleton, twins, and triplets or more are in parentheses.
Note: In rare cases a single embryo may divide and thus produce twins. For this reason, a small percentage of twins resulted from a single embryo transfer, and a small percentage of triplets resulted when two embryos were transferred.
†Total does not equal 100% due to rounding.

Appendix B

is just as, if not more, important in predicting success as the number of embryos transferred. Additionally, younger women tend to have both higher success rates and higher likelihood of multiple-infant births. Figure 34 shows the relationship between the number of embryos transferred, success rates, and multiple-infant births for a subset of ART procedures in which the woman was younger than 35 and the couple chose to set aside some embryos for future cycles rather than transfer all available embryos at one time.

For this group, the chance for a live birth using ART was about 49% when only one embryo was transferred. If one measures success as the percentage of transfers resulting in singleton live births, the highest likelihood of live birth was observed with only one embryo transferred.

The proportion of live births that were multiple-infant births was about 39% with two embryos and about 46% with three embryos. Transferring three or more embryos also created an additional risk for higher-order multiple births (i.e., triplets or more).

How long after egg retrieval does embryo transfer occur?

Once an ART cycle has progressed from egg retrieval to fertilization, the embryo(s) can be transferred into the woman's uterus in the subsequent 1 to 6 days. Figure 35 shows that in 2006 approximately 64% of embryo transfers occurred on day 3. Day 5 embryo transfers were the next most common, accounting for about 27% of ART procedures that progressed to the embryo transfer stage.

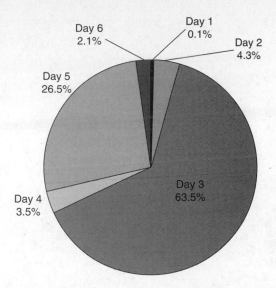

Figure 35   Day of Embryo Transfer* Among ART Cycles Using Fresh Nondonor Eggs or Embryos,† 2006.

*Number of days following egg retrieval.
†Cycles using GIFT or ZIFT are excluded. Missing or implausible values for day of embryo transfer (i.e., 0 or >6) are not included.

In general, is an ART cycle more likely to be successful if embryos are transferred on day 5?

As shown in Figure 35 (see above), in the vast majority of ART procedures, embryos were transferred on day 3 (64%) or day 5 (27%). Figure 36 compares success rates for day 3 embryo transfers with those for day 5 embryo transfers. In all age groups, the success rates were higher for day 5 embryo transfers than for day 3 transfers. However, some cycles do not progress to the embryo transfer stage because of embryo arrest (interruption in embryo development) between day 3 and day 5. These cycles are not accounted for in the success rates for day 5 transfers. Therefore, differences in success rates for day 3 and day 5 transfers should be interpreted with caution.

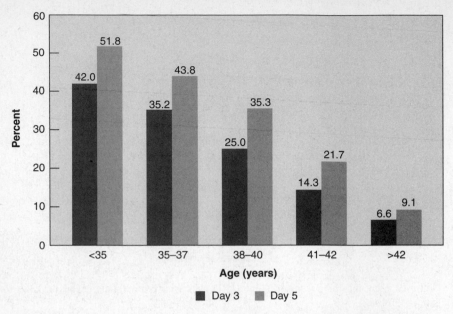

Figure 36   Percentages of Day 3 and Day 5 Embryo Transfers (Using Fresh Nondonor Eggs or Embryos) That Resulted in Live Births, by Woman's Age,* 2006.

*Cycles using GIFT or ZIFT are excluded. This comparison is limited to transfers on day 3 and day 5. Embryo transfers performed on days 1, 2, 4, and 6 are not included because each of these accounted for a small proportion of procedures.

Does the number of embryos transferred differ for day 3 and day 5 embryo transfers?

Figure 37 shows the number of embryos transferred on day 3 and day 5. Overall, fewer embryos were transferred on day 5 than on day 3. Approximately 53% of day 3 embryo transfers and 21% of day 5 embryo transfers involved the transfer of three or more embryos. The decrease in the number of embryos transferred on day 5, however, did not translate into a lower risk for multiple-infant births. See Figure 38 (page 222) for more details on the relationship between multiple-infant birth risk and day of embryo transfer.

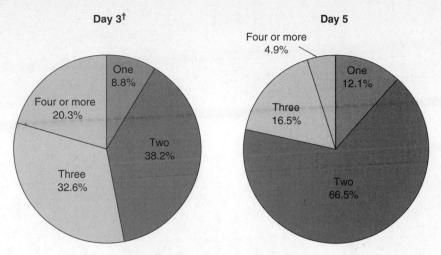

Figure 37   Number of Embryos Transferred During ART Cycles Using Fresh Nondonor Eggs or Embryos for Day 3 and Day 5 Embryo Transfers,* 2006.

*Cycles using GIFT or ZIFT are excluded. This comparison is limited to transfers on day 3 and day 5. Embryo transfers performed on days 1, 2, 4, and 6 are not included because each of these accounted for a small proportion of procedures.
†Total does not equal 100% due to rounding.

In general, how does the multiple-infant birth risk vary by the day of embryo transfer?

Multiple-infant births are associated with greater problems for both mothers and infants, including higher rates of caesarean section, prematurity, low birth weight, and infant disability or death.

Part A of Figure 38 shows that among the 16,519 live births that occurred following day 3 embryo transfer, 71% were singletons, 27% were twins, and about 2% were triplets or more. Thus, approximately 29% of these live births produced more than one infant.

In 2006, 9,567 live births occurred following day 5 embryo transfer. Part B of Figure 38 shows that 35% of these live births produced more than one infant (approximately 33% twins and 2% triplets or more).

As shown in Figure 37 (see above), fewer embryos were transferred on day 5 than on day 3. While the reduction in the number of embryos

221

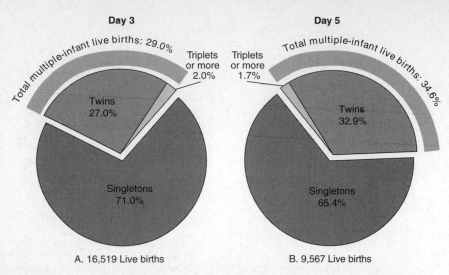

Figure 38   Risks of Having Multiple-Infant Live Birth for ART Cycles Using Fresh Nondonor Eggs or Embryos for Day 3 and Day 5 Embryo Transfers,* 2006.

*Cycles using GIFT or ZIFT are excluded. This comparison is limited to transfers on day 3 and day 5. Embryo transfers performed on days 1, 2, 4, and 6 are not included because each of these accounted for a small proportion of procedures.

transferred on day 5 was associated with a decrease in triplet-or-more births, it also was associated with an increase in twin births. Thus, the risk of having a multiple-infant birth was higher for day 5 embryo transfers. The likelihood of multiple-infant births for both day 3 and day 5 embryo transfers is much higher overall than for multiple-infant births in the general U.S. population (about 3%).

For day 5 embryo transfers, are success rates affected by the number of embryos transferred for women who have more embryos available than they choose to transfer?

As shown in Figure 37 (page 221), embryos transferred on day 5 result in more multiple-infant births compared with embryos transferred on day 3, despite the smaller number of embryos transferred on day 5. Figure 39 shows the relationship between the number of embryos transferred, the percentage of transfers resulting in live births, and the percentage of multiple-infant births for day 5 embryo transfer

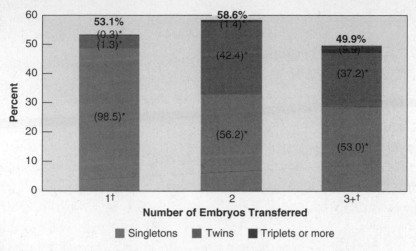

Figure 39   Percentages of Transfers That Resulted in Live Births and Percentages of Multiple-Infant Live Births for Day 5 Embryo Transfers Among Women Who Were Younger Than 35, Used Fresh Nondonor Eggs or Embryos, and Set Aside Extra Embryos for Future Use, by Number of Embryos Transferred, 2006.

*Percentages of live births that were singletons, twins, and triplets or more are in parentheses.
Note: In rare cases a single embryo may divide and thus produce twins. For this reason a small percentage of twins resulted from a single embryo transfer and a small percentage of triplets resulted when two embryos were transferred.
†Totals do not equal 100% due to rounding.

procedures in which the woman was younger than 35 and the couple decided to set aside some embryos for future cycles rather than transfer all available embryos at one time.

The percentage of transfers resulting in live births was 53% when only one embryo was transferred on day 5. The percentage of transfers resulting in live births was higher (59%) when two embryos were transferred; however, the proportion of live births that were multiples (twins or more)—which presents a higher risk for poor health outcomes—was 44%. The chance for a live birth was lower (50%) when 3 or more embryos were transferred on day 5, and the percentage of live births that were higher-order multiples (triplets or more) was much higher for these transfers (10%) than for those involving the transfer of just two embryos on day 5 (1.4%).

If one measures success as the percentage of transfers resulting in singleton live births, the highest rate (53%) was observed with the transfer of a single embryo on day 5.

What are the success rates for women who use gestational carriers?

In some cases a woman has trouble carrying a pregnancy. In such cases the couple may use ART with a gestational carrier, sometimes called a surrogate. A gestational carrier is a woman who agrees to carry the developing embryo for a couple with infertility problems. Gestational carriers were used in 1% of ART cycles using fresh nondonor embryos in 2006 (1,042 cycles). Figure 40 compares success rates per transfer for ART cycles that used a gestational carrier in 2006 with cycles that did not. In all age groups,

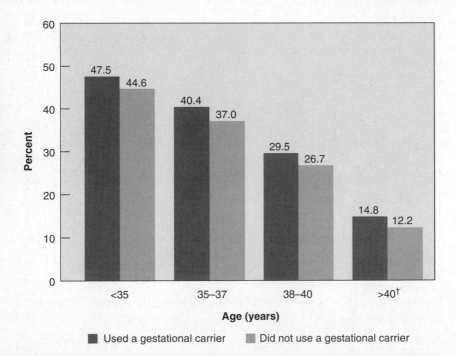

Figure 40   Comparison of Percentages of Transfers That Resulted in Live Births Between Cycles That Used Gestational Carriers and Those That Did Not (Both Using Fresh Nondonor Embryos), by ART Patient's Age,* 2006.

*Age categories reflect the age of the ART patient, not the age of the gestational carrier.
†We were unable to further subdivide ages >40 because the number of such cycles is very small.

success rates for ART cycles that used gestational carriers were higher than success rates for those cycles that did not.

How is clinic size related to success rates?

The number of ART procedures carried out every year varies among fertility clinics in the United States. In 2006, success rates were similar for all 426 clinics regardless of the number of cycles performed. For Figure 41, clinics were divided equally into four groups (called quartiles) based on the size of the clinic as determined by the number of cycles it carried out. The percentage for each quartile represents the average success rate for clinics in that quartile.

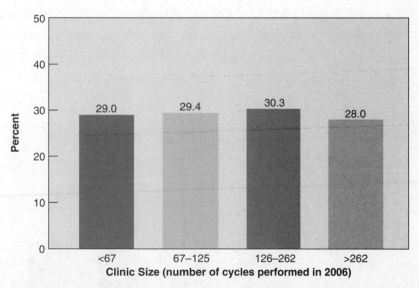

Figure 41   Percentages of ART Cycles (Using Fresh Nondonor Eggs or Embryos) That Resulted in Live Births, by Clinic Size, 2006.

SECTION 3: ART CYCLES USING FROZEN NONDONOR EMBRYOS

What are the success rates for ART cycles using frozen nondonor embryos?

Frozen embryos were used in approximately 16% of all ART cycles performed in 2006 (22,023 cycles). Figure 42 compares the success rates for frozen embryos with the success rates for fresh embryos among women using their own eggs. Because some embryos do not survive the thawing process, the percentage of thawed embryos that result in live births is usually lower than the percentage of transfers resulting in live births. In 2006, the success rates for frozen embryos were lower than the success rates for fresh embryos. However, the average number of embryos transferred was similar for cycles using both frozen embryos and fresh embroys. It is important to note that cycles using frozen embryos are both less expensive and less invasive than those using fresh embryos because the

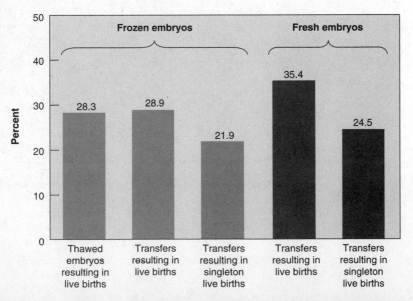

Figure 42   Success Rates for ART Cycles Using Frozen Embryos and Fresh Embryos, 2006.

woman does not have to go through the fertility drug stimulation and egg retrieval steps again.

What is the risk of having a multiple-fetus pregnancy or multiple-infant live birth from an ART cycle using frozen nondonor embryos?

Multiple-infant births are associated with greater problems for both mothers and infants, including higher rates of caesarean section, prematurity, low birth weight, and infant disability or death.

Part A of Figure 43 shows that among the 7,401 pregnancies that resulted from ART cycles using frozen nondonor embryos, 66% were singleton pregnancies, 21% were twins, and 3% were triplets or more. Ten percent of pregnancies ended in miscarriage before the number of fetuses could be accurately determined. Therefore, the percentage of pregnancies with more than one fetus might have been higher than what was reported (24%).

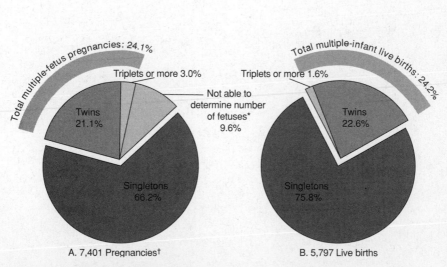

Figure 43   Risks of Having Multiple-Fetus Pregnancy and Multiple-Infant Live Birth from ART Cycles Using Frozen Nondonor Embryos, 2006.

*Number of fetuses not known because the pregnancy ended in an early miscarriage.
†Total does not equal 100% due to rounding.

In 2006, 5,797 pregnancies from ART cycles that used frozen non-donor embryos resulted in live births. Part B of Figure 43 shows that approximately 24% of these live births produced more than one infant. This compares with a multiple-infant birth rate of slightly more than 3% in the general U.S. population.

Although the total rates for multiples were similar for pregnancies and live births, there were more triplet-or-more pregnancies than births. Triplet-or-more pregnancies may be reduced to twins or singletons by the time of birth. This can happen naturally (e.g., fetal death), or a woman and her doctor may decide to reduce the number of fetuses using a procedure called multifetal pregnancy reduction. CDC does not collect information on multifetal pregnancy reductions.

SECTION 4: ART CYCLES USING DONOR EGGS

Are older women undergoing ART more likely to use donor eggs or embryos?

As shown in Figures 14–16 (pages 196–198), eggs produced by women in older age groups form embryos that are less likely to implant and more likely to result in miscarriage if they do implant. As a result, ART using donor eggs is much more common among older women than among younger women. Donor eggs or embryos were used in approximately 12% of all ART cycles carried out in 2006 (16,976 cycles). Figure 44 shows the percentage of ART cycles using donor eggs in 2006 according to the woman's age. Few women younger than age 39 used donor eggs; however, the percentage of cycles carried out with donor eggs increased sharply starting at age 39. Among women older than age 47, for example, about 89% of all ART cycles used donor eggs.

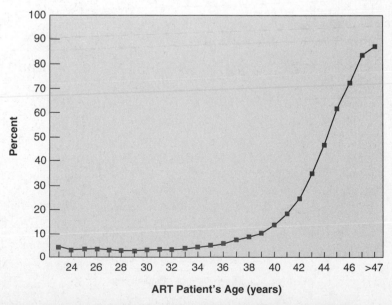

Figure 44   Percentage of ART Cycles Using Donor Eggs, by ART Patient's Age, 2006.

Do success rates differ by age for women who used ART with donor eggs compared with women who used ART with their own eggs?

Figure 45 compares percentages of transfers resulting in live births for ART cycles using fresh embryos from donor eggs with those for ART cycles using a woman's own eggs, among women of different ages. The likelihood of a fertilized egg implanting is related to the age of the woman who produced the egg. Thus, the percentage of transfers resulting in live births for cycles using embryos from women's own eggs declines as women get older. In contrast, since egg donors are typically in their 20s or early 30s, the percentage of transfers resulting in live births for cycles using embryos from donor eggs remained consistently high at above 40%.

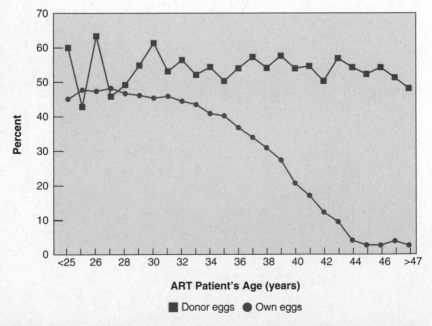

Figure 45   Percentages of Transfers That Resulted in Live Births for ART Cycles Using Fresh Embryos from Own and Donor Eggs, by ART Patient's Age, 2006.

How successful is ART when donor eggs are used?

Figure 46 shows percentages of transfers resulting in live births and singleton live births for ART cycles using fresh embryos from donor eggs among women of different ages. For all ages, the percentage of transfers resulting in singleton live births (average 33%) was lower than the percentage of transfers resulting in live births (average 54%). Singleton live births are an important measure of success because they have a much lower risk than multiple-infant births for adverse infant health outcomes, including prematurity, low birth weight, disability, and death.

Appendix B

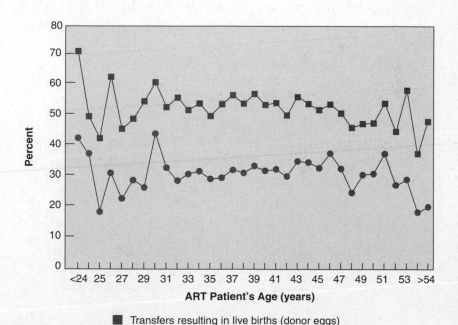

Figure 46   Percentages of Transfers That Resulted in Live Births and Singleton Live Births for ART Cycles Using Fresh Embryos from Donor Eggs, by ART Patient's Age, 2006.

What is the risk of having a multiple-fetus pregnancy or multiple-infant live birth from an ART cycle using fresh donor eggs?

Multiple-infant births are associated with greater problems for both mothers and infants, including higher rates of caesarean section, prematurity, low birth weight, and infant disability or death.

Part A of Figure 47 shows that among the 6,315 pregnancies that resulted from ART cycles using fresh embryos from donor eggs, about 54% were singleton pregnancies, about 37% were twins, and nearly 4% were triplets or more. About 5% of pregnancies ended in miscarriage before the number of fetuses could be accurately determined. Therefore, the percentage of pregnancies with more than one fetus might have been higher than what was reported (about 41%).

In 2006, 5,393 pregnancies from ART cycles that used fresh embryos from donor eggs resulted in live births. Part B of Figure 47 shows that 39% of these live births produced more than one infant.

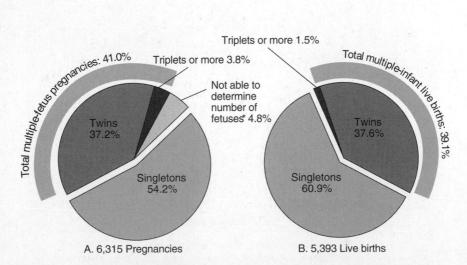

Figure 47   Risks of Having Multiple-Fetus Pregnancy and Multiple-Infant Live Birth from ART Cycles Using Fresh Embryos from Donor Eggs, 2006.

*Number of fetuses not known because the pregnancy ended in an early miscarriage.

This compares with a multiple-infant birth rate of slightly more than 3% in the general population.

Although the total rates for multiples were similar for pregnancies and live births, there were more triplet-or-more pregnancies than births. Triplet-or-more pregnancies may be reduced to twins or singletons by the time of birth. This can happen naturally (e.g., fetal death), or a woman and her doctor may decide to reduce the number of fetuses using a procedure called multifetal pregnancy reduction. CDC does not collect information on multifetal pregnancy reductions.

How do success rates differ between women who use frozen donor embryos and those who use fresh donor embryos?

Figure 48 shows that the success rates resulting from the transfer of frozen donor embryos were substantially lower than the success

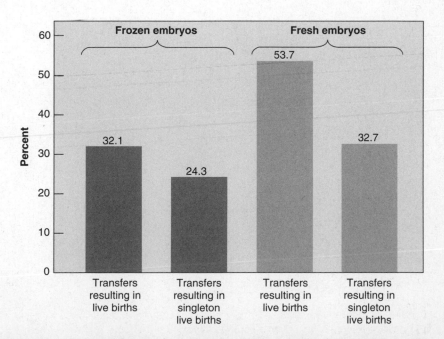

Figure 48   Success Rates for ART Cycles Using Frozen Donor and Fresh Donor Embryos, 2006.

rates resulting from the transfer of fresh donor embryos. This is similar to the findings for frozen nondonor embryos (see Figure 42, page 226). The average number of embryos transferred was similar for cycles using frozen donor embryos and those using fresh donor embryos.

SECTION 5: ART TRENDS, 1996–2006

This report marks the twelfth consecutive year that CDC has published an annual report detailing the success rates for ART clinics in the United States. Having several years of data provides us with the opportunity to examine trends in ART use and success rates over time. Because the first year of data collection, 1995, did not include non-SART member clinics, we limit our examination of trends to the years 1996–2006.

Is the use of ART increasing?

Figure 49 shows the numbers of ART cycles performed, live-birth deliveries, and infants born using ART from 1996 through 2006. The number of ART cycles performed in the United States has more than doubled, from 64,681 cycles in 1996 to 138,198 in 2006. The number of live-birth deliveries in 2006 (41,343) was more than two and a half times higher than in 1996 (14,507). The number of infants born who were conceived using ART also increased steadily between 1996 and 2006. In 2006, 54,656 infants were born, which

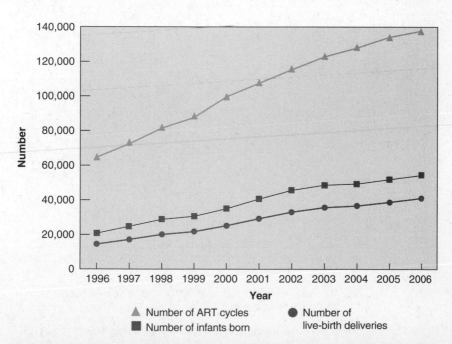

Figure 49   Numbers of ART Cycles Performed, Live-Birth Deliveries, and Infants Born Using ART, 1996–2006.

was more than two and a half times the 20,840 born in 1996. Because in some cases more than one infant is born during a live-birth delivery (e.g., twins), the total number of infants born is greater than the number of live-birth deliveries.

Have there been changes in the type of ART cycles performed among women who used fresh or frozen nondonor eggs or embryos?

Intracytoplasmic sperm injection (ICSI) was originally developed to use in ART cycles to improve fertilization rates when severe male factor infertility was the indication for using ART. Today, this procedure is widely used even among couples without a diagnosis of male factor infertility.

Figure 50 shows the numbers of ART cycles performed using fresh nondonor eggs or embryos with or without ICSI and the numbers of

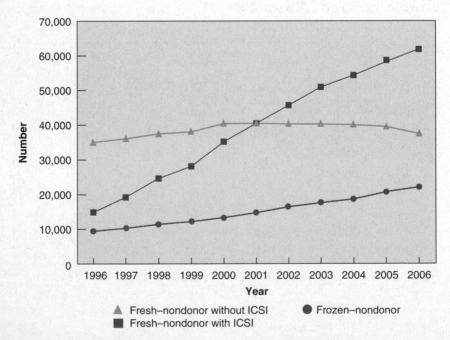

Figure 50   Numbers of ART Cycles Using Fresh or Frozen Nondonor Eggs or Embryos, by ICSI,* 1996–2006.

*Intracytoplasmic sperm injection.

cycles using frozen nondonor eggs or embryos from 1996 through 2006. During the past 11 years, while the number of fresh–nondonor cycles performed without ICSI remained stable, the number of fresh–nondonor cycles performed with ICSI increased four times from 14,885 in 1996 to 61,835 in 2006. The number of frozen–nondonor cycles more than doubled, from 9,445 in 1996 to 22,023 in 2006.

Note that the information on use of ICSI was not collected for ART cycles using frozen embryos; therefore, cycles using frozen embryos are presented together as one group.

Have there been changes in the types of ART cycles performed among women who used fresh or frozen donor eggs or embryos?

Figure 51 shows the numbers of ART cycles performed using fresh donor eggs or embryos with or without ICSI and cycles using

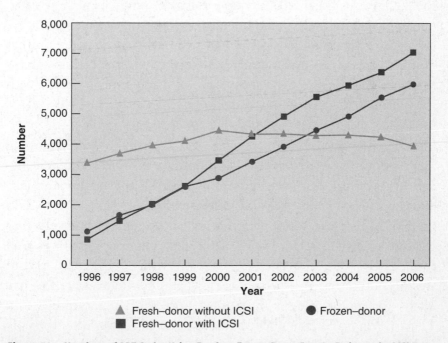

Figure 51   Numbers of ART Cycles Using Fresh or Frozen Donor Eggs or Embryos, by ICSI,* 1996–2006.

*Intracytoplasmic sperm injection.

frozen donor eggs or embryos. While the number of fresh–donor cycles performed without ICSI remained fairly stable during the past 11 years, the number of fresh–donor cycles performed with ICSI increased from 857 in 1996 to 7,039 in 2006. The number of frozen–donor cycles increased from 1,118 in 1996 to 5,992 in 2006. In particular, during reporting year 2006, fresh donor eggs with ICSI were used the most among all donor cycles.

Note that the information on use of ICSI was not collected for ART cycles using frozen embryos; therefore, cycles using frozen embryos are presented together as one group.

Have there been improvements in the percentage of transfers that result in live births among women who used fresh or frozen nondonor eggs or embryos?

Figure 52 presents percentages of transfers that resulted in live births for ART cycles using fresh nondonor eggs or embryos with or without ICSI and for cycles using frozen nondonor eggs or embryos. Percentages of transfers that resulted in live births are presented rather than percentages of cycles that resulted in live births because this is the only way to directly compare cycles using fresh embryos with those using frozen embryos.

Overall, higher success rates were consistently observed among fresh–nondonor cycles than frozen–nondonor cycles. The percentage of transfers that resulted in live births for fresh–nondonor cycles performed without ICSI increased from 28% in 1996 to 37% in 2006. Over the same period, the percentage of transfers that resulted in live births for cycles using fresh nondonor embryos performed with ICSI remained slightly lower than without ICSI, but steadily increased. The percentage of transfers that resulted in live births for cycles using frozen nondonor embryos increased from 17% in 1996 to 29% in 2006, but was generally lower than the percentage of transfers that resulted in live births for cycles using fresh nondonor embryos.

Appendix B

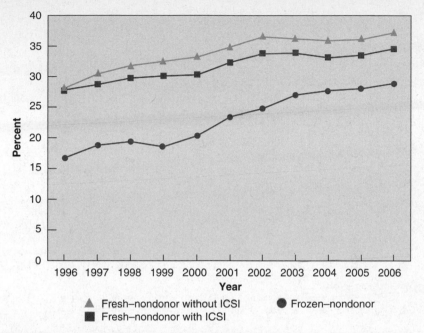

Figure 52   Percentages of Transfers That Resulted in Live Births Using Fresh or Frozen Nondonor Eggs or Embryos, by ICSI,* 1996–2006.

*Intracytoplasmic sperm injection.

Note that the information on use of ICSI was not collected for ART cycles using frozen embryos; therefore, such cycles are presented together as one group.

Have there been improvements in the percentage of transfers that result in live births among women who used fresh or frozen donor eggs or embryos?

Figure 53 presents the percentages of transfers that resulted in live births for ART cycles using fresh donor eggs or embryos with or without ICSI and for cycles using frozen donor eggs or embryos. Percentages of transfers that resulted in live births are presented rather than percentages of cycles that resulted in live births because that is the only way to directly compare cycles using fresh embryos with those using frozen embryos.

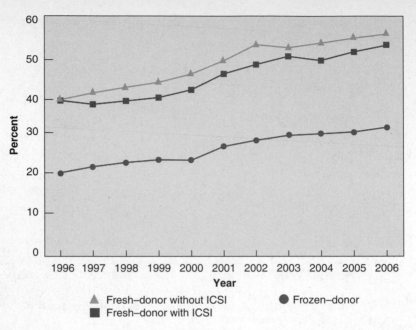

Figure 53   Percentages of Transfers That Resulted in Live Births Using Fresh or Frozen Donor Eggs or Embryos, by ICSI,* 1996–2006.

*Intracytoplasmic sperm injection.

Similar to the trends shown in Figure 52 (page 239) for nondonor cycles, the success rates for cycles using fresh donor eggs or embryos were generally higher than for cycles using frozen donor eggs or embryos during 1996–2006. The percentage of transfers that resulted in live births for cycles that used fresh donor eggs or embryos performed without ICSI increased from 39% in 1996 to 56% in 2006. Over the same period, the percentage of transfers resulting in live births increased from 39% to 53% for cycles that used fresh donor eggs or embryos and were performed with ICSI, and from 21% to 32% for cycles that used frozen donor eggs or embryos.

Note that the information on use of ICSI was not collected for ART cycles using frozen embryos; therefore, such cycles are presented together as one group.

Have there been improvements in the percentage of transfers that result in singleton live births among women who used fresh or frozen nondonor eggs or embryos?

Singleton live births are an important measure of success because they entail a much lower risk than multiple-infant births for adverse infant health outcomes, including prematurity, low birth weight, disability, and death. Figure 54 presents percentages of transfers that resulted in singleton live births for ART cycles performed using fresh nondonor eggs or embryos with or without ICSI or for cycles using frozen nondonor eggs or embryos.

While the total numbers of nondonor cycles using ICSI greatly increased over the past 11 years (see Figure 50, page 236), the

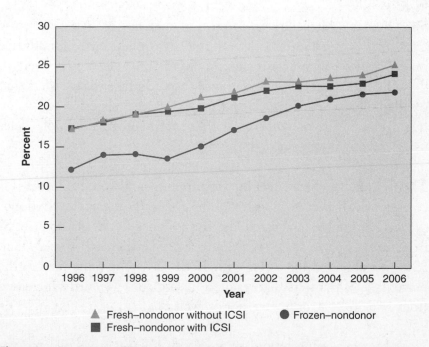

Figure 54   Percentages of Transfers That Resulted in Singleton Live Births Among Women Using Fresh or Frozen Nondonor Eggs or Embryos, by ICSI,* 1996–2006.

*Intracytoplasmic sperm injection.

percentage of transfers that resulted in singleton live births from these cycles was not any higher than those without ICSI: 17% to 24% with ICSI versus 17% to 25% without ICSI.

Over the same period, the percentage of transfers that resulted in singleton live births among frozen–nondonor cycles increased from 12% to 22%.

Note that the information on use of ICSI was not collected for ART cycles using frozen embryos; therefore, such cycles are presented together as one group.

Have there been improvements in the percentage of transfers that result in singleton live births among women who used fresh or frozen donor eggs or embryos?

Singleton live births are an important measure of success because they entail a much lower risk than multiple-infant births for adverse infant health outcomes, including prematurity, low birth weight, disability, and death. Figure 55 presents percentages of transfers that resulted in singleton live births for ART cycles performed using fresh donor eggs or embryos with or without ICSI or for cycles using frozen donor eggs or embryos.

The percentage of transfers that resulted in singleton live births was consistently higher for fresh–donor cycles than for frozen–donor cycles. Percentages increased for fresh–donor cycles without ICSI from 22% in 1996 to 33% in 2006; a similar increase from 24% to 33% was observed for cycles with ICSI. Over the same period, the percentage of transfers that resulted in singleton live births increased from 15% to 24% for frozen–donor cycles.

Note that the information on use of ICSI was not collected for ART cycles using frozen embryos; therefore, such cycles are presented together as one group.

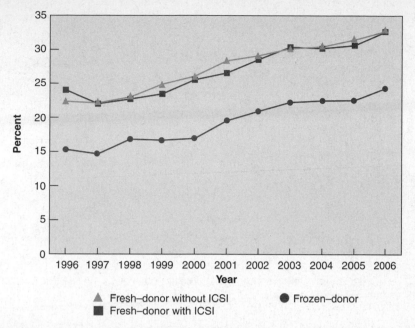

Figure 55   Percentages of Transfers That Resulted in Singleton Live Births Among Women Using Fresh or Frozen Donor Eggs or Embryos, by ICSI,* 1996–2006.

*Intracytoplasmic sperm injection.

Have there been improvements in the percentage of transfers that result in live births for all ART patients or only for those in particular age groups?

Figure 56 presents percentages of transfers that resulted in live births, by woman's age, for ART cycles using fresh nondonor eggs or embryos.

From 1996 through 2006, the percentage of transfers that resulted in live births for women younger than 35 increased 33%, from 34% in 1996 to 45% in 2006. Over the same period, the percentage of transfers that resulted in live births increased 28% for women 35–37, 24% for women 38–40, 31% for women 41–42, and 22% for women older than 42.

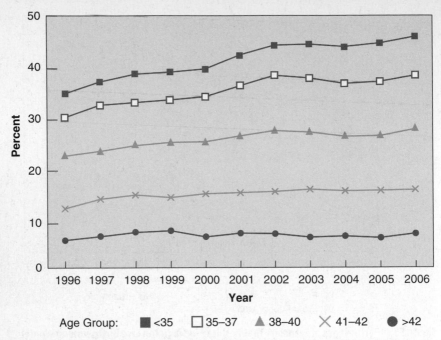

Figure 56   Percentages of Transfers That Resulted in Live Births for ART Cycles Using Fresh Nondonor Eggs or Embryos, by Woman's Age, 1996–2006.

Have there been improvements in the percentage of transfers that result in singleton live births for all ART patients or only for those in particular age groups?

Singleton live births are an important measure of success because they have a much lower risk than multiple-infant births for adverse infant health outcomes, including prematurity, low birth weight, disability, and death. Figure 57 presents percentages of transfers that resulted in singleton live births, by woman's age, for ART cycles using fresh nondonor eggs or embryos.

From 1996 through 2006, the percentage of transfers that resulted in singleton live births for women younger than 35 increased about 52%, from 19% in 1996 to 29% in 2006. Over the same period, the

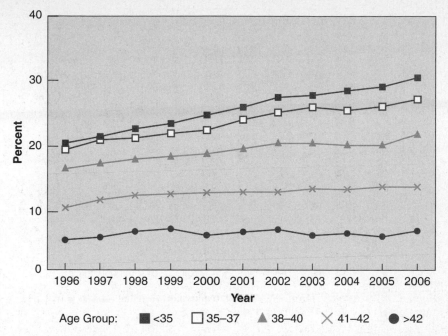

Figure 57   Percentages of Transfers (Using Fresh Nondonor Eggs or Embryos) That Resulted in Singleton Live Births, by Woman's Age, 1996–2006.

percentage of transfers that resulted in singleton live births increased 42% for women 35–37, 34% for women 38–40, 34% for women 41–42, and 30% for women older than 42.

Has the number of embryos transferred in fresh–nondonor cycles changed?

Figure 58 presents the trends for number of embryos transferred in fresh–nondonor cycles that progressed to the embryo transfer stage. From 1996 through 2006, cycles that involved the transfer of one embryo increased slightly, from 6% to 11%; cycles that involved the transfer of two embryos increased dramatically, from 10% in 1996 to 46% in 2006. Cycles that involved the transfer of three embryos increased from 23% in 1996 to 28% in 2006, and cycles that involved the transfer of four or more embryos decreased from 62% in 1996 to 16% in 2006.

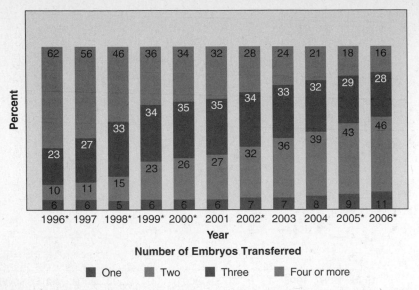

Figure 58   Percentages of Fresh–Nondonor Cycles That Involved the Transfer of One, Two, Three, or Four or More Embryos, 1996–2006.

*Totals do not equal 100% due to rounding.

Has the number of embryos transferred in each ART cycle changed for women younger than 35 who have more embryos available than they choose to transfer?

As shown in Figure 58 (see above), the number of embryos transferred in fresh–nondonor cycles has decreased during the past 11 years. Figure 59 shows the change over time in the number of embryos transferred for ART procedures in which the woman was younger than 35 and the couple chose to set aside some embryos for future cycles rather than transfer all available embryos at one time. Previous research suggests that the number of embryos available for an ART cycle is important in predicting success. Younger women also tend to have higher success rates (see Figure 14, page 196).

Overall, the number of embryos transferred decreased among couples who chose to transfer fewer embryos than were available. In 1996, almost two-thirds (64%) of ART cycles involved the transfer of four or more embryos; 33%, three embryos; 3%, two embryos; and less than 1%, one embryo. By 1998, the percentage of cycles in

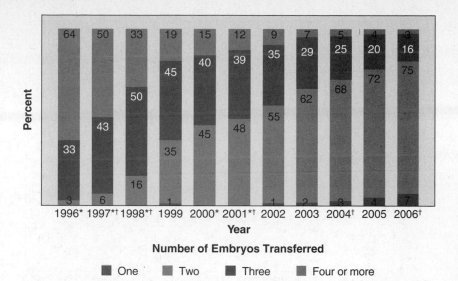

Figure 59   Percentages of Fresh–Nondonor Cycles That Involved the Transfer of One, Two, Three, or Four or More Embryos in Women Who Were Younger Than 35 and Set Aside Extra Embryos for Future Use, 1996–2006.

*Cycles involving the transfer of one embryo were not included because of the small number of cycles where one embryo was transferred and extra embryos were set aside for future use.
†Totals do not equal 100% due to rounding.

which four or more embryos were transferred had decreased to 33%; half of all ART cycles involved the transfer of three embryos; 16% of cycles, two embryos; and less than 1%, one embryo. By 2006, four or more embryos were transferred in only 3% of cycles, three in 16% of cycles, two in 75% of cycles, and one in 7% of cycles.

Have there been improvements in ART success rates, by number of embryos transferred?

Figure 60 presents success rates by the number of embryos transferred for ART cycles using fresh nondonor eggs or embryos from 1996 through 2006. In general, success rates were higher when two or more embryos were transferred. From 1996 through 2006, the success rates tripled, from 14% to 42%, for ART cycles that involved the transfer of two embryos. The success rates also increased for ART cycles that involved the transfer of either one or three embryos; however, the success rates decreased 13%, from 32% to 28%, for ART cycles that involved the transfer of four or more embryos.

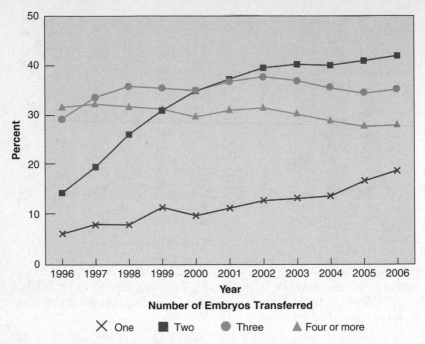

Figure 60   Percentages of Transfers (Using Fresh Nondonor Eggs or Embryos) That Resulted in Live Births, by Number of Embryos Transferred, 1996–2006.

The relationship between number of embryos transferred and success rates is complicated by several factors, such as the woman's age and embryo quality. Trends over time may reflect changes in these factors.

Have there been improvements in the percentage of transfers that resulted in live births for women younger than 35 who have more embryos available than they choose to transfer?

Figure 61 shows changes over time in the number of embryos transferred and the percentage of transfers that resulted in live births for ART cycles in which the woman was younger than 35 and chose to set aside some embryos for future cycles rather than transfer all available embryos at one time. Previous research suggests that the number of embryos available for an ART cycle is an important predictor of success. Younger women also tend to have higher success rates (see Figure 14, page 196).

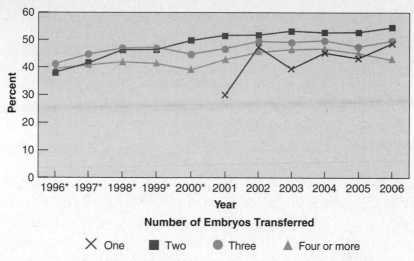

Number of Embryos Transferred

X One ■ Two ● Three ▲ Four or more

Figure 61   Percentages of Transfers That Resulted in Live Births Among Women Who Were Younger Than 35 and Set Aside Extra Embryos for Future Use, by Number of Embryos Transferred, 1996–2006.

*Cycles involving the transfer of one embryo were not included because of the small number of cycles where one embryo was transferred and extra embryos were set aside for future use.

For this group of women, the percentage of transfers that resulted in live births generally increased over time, regardless of the number of embryos transferred. The biggest increase was for cycles in which two embryos were transferred. In 1996, the chance for a live birth was highest (41%) when three embryos were transferred; however, in 2006, the chance for a live birth was highest (55%) when two embryos were transferred.

Success rates for cycles involving the transfer of one embryo were comparable to those that involved multiple embryos. Elective single-embryo transfer minimizes the risk for multiple-infant pregnancy and related adverse outcomes. Recently, the Society for Assisted Reproductive Technology (SART) revised its embryo transfer guidelines to encourage single-embryo transfer among patients with good prognoses.**

**For more information, contact SART (by telephone at 205-978-5000 or online at www.sart.org).

Appendix B

Has the percentage of multiple-infant live births changed?

Multiple-infant births are associated with greater problems for both mothers and infants, including higher rates of caesarean section, prematurity, low birth weight, and infant disability or death. Figure 62 shows the percentages of multiple-infant live births for the four primary types of ART procedures.

For fresh–nondonor cycles, the percentage of multiple-infant live births decreased 20% since 1996, from 38% of all live births in 1996 to 31% in 2006. Over the same period, the percentage of multiple-infant live births decreased 10% for frozen–nondonor cycles and 6% for fresh–donor cycles. In all years except 1997, the percentage of multiple-infant live births remained stable for frozen–donor cycles.

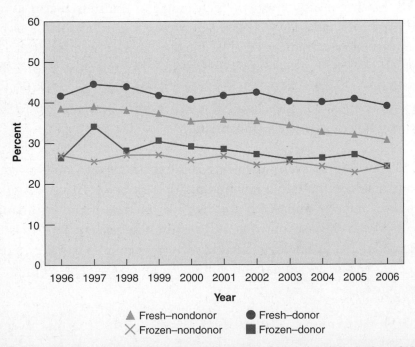

Figure 62   Percentages of Cycles That Resulted in Multiple-Infant Live Births, by Type of ART Cycle, 1996–2006.

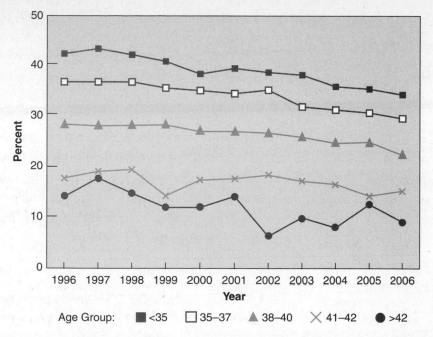

Age Group: ■ <35   ☐ 35–37   ▲ 38–40   ✕ 41–42   ● >42

Figure 63 **Percentages of Multiple-Infant Live Births, for Fresh–Nondonor Cycles, by ART Patient's Age, 1996–2006.**

Have multiple-infant live births for cycles using fresh nondonor eggs or embryos changed for all ART patients or only for those in particular age groups?

Figure 63 shows that the percentages of multiple-infant live births decreased between 1996 and 2006 for women in all age groups. In 1996, 43% of live-birth deliveries to women younger than 35 were multiple-infant births, compared with 34% in 2006. Among women older than 42, the percentages of multiple-infant live births decreased from 14% in 1996 to 9% in 2006.

Have the percentages of singletons, twins, and triplets or more changed for ART cycles using fresh nondonor eggs or embryos?

Figure 64 presents the trends in percentages of transfers that resulted in live births and percentages of multiple-infant live births for ART cycles using fresh nondonor eggs or embryos. Overall, the percentage of transfers that resulted in live births increased from 28% in 1996 to 35% in 2006. From 1996 through 2006, the percentage of singleton live births increased from 62% to 69%; the percentage of twin births remained stable, ranging from 29% to 32%; and the percentage of triplet-or-more births decreased from 7% in 1996 to 2% in 2006.

It is important to note that twins, albeit to a lesser extent than triplets or more, are still at substantially greater risk for illness and death than singletons. These risks include low birth weight, preterm birth, and neurological impairments such as cerebral palsy. Both the percentages of twin and triplet-or-more births remain significantly higher for ART births than for births resulting from natural conception.

Courtesy of Centers for Disease Control and Prevention, American Society for Reproductive Medicine, Society for Assisted Reproductive Technology. 2006 Assisted Reproductive Technology Success Rates: National Summary and Fertility Clinic Reports, Atlanta: U.S. Department of Health and Human Services, Centers for Disease Control and Prevention; 2008.

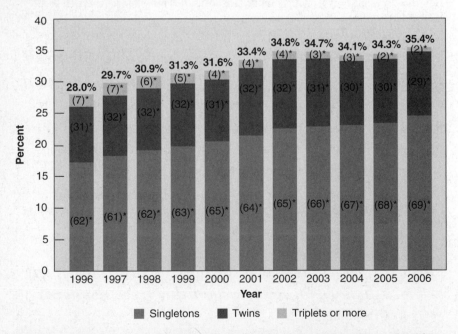

Figure 64   Percentages of Transfers That Resulted in Live Births and Percentages of Multiple-Infant Live Births for ART Cycles Using Fresh Nondonor Eggs or Embryos, 1996–2006.

*Percentages of live births that were singletons, twins, and triplets or more are in parentheses.
†Total does not equal 100% due to rounding.

Glossary

A

Acanthosis nigricans: A velvety skin discoloration associated with insulin resistance.

Acrosome reaction: A test to assess the biochemical changes on the head of the sperm that may predict the ability of the sperm to fertilize an egg.

Adhesions: Bands of fibrous tissue that can bind reproductive organs, thereby reducing a woman's fertility.

Aneuploidy: Having an abnormal number of chromosomes.

Anovulation: Failure to release an egg on a regular basis, resulting in irregular or absent periods.

Anticardiolipin antibodies: Specific antibodies that are formed against various components of the cells of the body; their presence is often associated with pregnancy loss.

Antimullerian hormone (AMH): A protein hormone that is used to evaluate a patient's ovarian reserve.

Antiphospholipid antibodies: The general class of antibodies that are formed against various components of the cells of the body; their presence is often associated with pregnancy loss.

Antisperm antibodies: Proteins that can lead to infertility by impairing fertilization or enhancing sperm destruction within the female reproductive tract.

Antithrombin III: A protein involved in the coagulation cascade. A deficiency in antithrombin III is associated with an increased risk of blood clotting and pregnancy loss.

Antral follicle count: The number of resting follicles seen on ultrasound early in a woman's cycle.

Artificial insemination: A group of fertility procedures involving the introduction of sperm into the female reproductive tract without intercourse.

Assisted hatching: The process of thining the outer shell of the embryo (zona pellucida) prior to embryo transfer to promote its implantation in the uterus.

Assisted reproductive technologies (ART): A variety of fertility procedures (including in vitro fertilization) that involve manipulating sperm and eggs to achieve pregnancy.

Autosomal dominant diseases: Genetic diseases carried on a chromosome other than the X or Y chromosomes (sex chromosomes), in which a single abnormal copy of the gene leads to the presence of the disease.

Autosomal recessive diseases: Genetic diseases carried on a chromosome other than the X or Y chromosomes (sex chromosomes), in which two abnormal copies of the gene are necessary for the disease to be present.

Azoospermia: The absence of sperm in a semen analysis.

B

Balanced translocation: A chromosomal rearrangement in which two chromosomes break apart and re-form as a new chromosome containing parts of both of the original chromosomes.

Blastocyst: A stage in embryo development reached 5 days after fertilization.

Blastomeres: The individual cells present in an early cleavage-stage embryo.

Body mass index (BMI): A mathematical calculation that uses height and weight to determine whether an individual is of normal weight, overweight, or obese.

C

Chlamydia: A common sexually transmitted disease that can damage a woman's fallopian tubes.

Chromosomes: One of the threadlike "packages" of genes and other DNA in the nucleus of a cell. Humans have 23 pairs of chromosomes, for a total of 46 in all: 44 autosomes and 2 sex chromosomes.

Clomiphene citrate challenge test (CCCT): A test used to evaluate a woman's ovarian reserve before she undergoes a fertility treatment.

Congenital bilateral absence of the vas deferens (CBAVD): Absence of the sperm-carrying duct in a man, resulting in azoospermia. This condition is frequently associated with cystic fibrosis.

Controlled ovarian hyperstimulation: Stimulation of the ovaries with fertility medications to help them grow and release multiple eggs.

Corpus luteum: The hormone-producing ovarian cyst that forms from the follicle after it releases the egg.

Cryopreservation: Freezing of sperm, eggs, or embryos so as to preserve them for use at a later date.

D

Day-3 hormones: Measurement of follicle-stimulating hormone and estradiol on the second or third day of a regular menstrual cycle, which provides an assessment of a woman's ovarian reserve.

Diminished ovarian reserve: The inability to respond appropriately to fertility medications, both in terms of the number of follicles produced and the health of the eggs.

Dizygotic twins: Twins resulting from the implantation of embryos from two different eggs (also called fraternal twins).

Donor-egg IVF: An extremely successful type of in vitro fertilization procedure using the eggs from a young woman and with the resulting embryo(s) transferred into the recipient.

Dysmenorrhea: Extremely painful periods.

E

Ectopic pregnancy: A pregnancy located outside the uterine cavity, usually in the fallopian tube, though it can also occur in the ovary or abdomen (rarely).

Egg collection: A minimally invasive procedure usually performed transvaginally under minimal sedation in which eggs are removed from the ovaries.

Embryo transfer: The placement of embryos created via in vitro fertilization into the uterus or, more rarely, the fallopian tube.

Embryologist: A scientist involved in the fertilization and culture of human eggs and embryos.

Endometrial biopsy: A sample of the lining of the uterus, usually performed to rule out endometrial cancer.

Endometriomas: An ovarian cyst that is filled with chocolate-colored fluid as a result of endometriosis growing within the ovary.

Endometriosis: The presence of tissue that is usually found within the endometrial cavity in another location (most frequently on the ovaries or along the uterosacral ligaments).

Endometrium: The tissue that lines the uterine cavity and is shed each month with a woman's period.

Epididymis: Paired sac-like structures that are found atop each testicle and that serve as a repository for sperm prior to ejaculation.

Estrogen: A steroid hormone produced within the growing follicle that induces growth of the endometrium.

F

Factor V Leiden: A genetic disorder that predisposes a woman to blood clot formation and miscarriage.

Fallopian tube: The conduit that serves as an incubator following release and fertilization of the egg.

Fertilization: The process by which an egg and a sperm combine and create an embryo.

Fibroids: Benign growths of the connective tissue of the uterus that can grow quite large and cause menstrual problems, infertility, and miscarriage.

Fifth's disease: An infectious disease caused by parvovirus B19. It leads to bright rosy checks in children but can cause miscarriage if a woman contracts it during pregnancy.

Fimbria: The finger-like projections at the distal end of the fallopian tube that are responsible for trapping the egg following ovulation.

Flare stimulation protocol: A technique of follicular stimulation that begins at the start of a spontaneous menstrual cycle.

Follicles: Fluid-filled structures within the ovary that contain an egg.

Follicle-stimulating hormone (FSH): A protein hormone produced within the pituitary gland at the base of the brain that promotes the growth and development of follicles, leading eventually to ovulation.

Frozen embryo transfer (FET): Placement of previously cryopreserved embryos into the uterus or, more rarely, the fallopian tube.

Functional hypothalamic amenorrhea (FHA): The absence of menstrual cycles related to failure of the hypothalamus and pituitary gland to stimulate follicular growth.

G

Gestational carrier: A woman who undergoes an embryo transfer consisting of an embryo produced by another couple (or from donor gametes) with the intention to give the resulting baby back to the genetic parents.

Gonadotropin-releasing hormone (GnRH) analog: Medication that initially causes the pituitary gland to release its stores of follicle-stimulating hormone and luteinizing hormone, but that with continued use leads to markedly suppressed levels of these two hormones.

Gonadotropin-releasing hormone (GnRH) antagonist: Medication that quickly interferes with the production of follicle-stimulating hormone and luteinizing hormone by the pituitary gland, preventing premature ovulation during a treatment cycle.

Gonadotropins: Fertility medications containing follicle-stimulating hormone alone or in combination with luteinizing hormone that are used to induce follicle growth during fertility treatments.

Gonorrhea: A sexually transmitted disease that can cause tubal damage and infertility.

H

Heparin: An injectable medication that is used to prevent blood clot formation.

Human chorionic gonadotropin (HCG): A placental hormone produced in pregnancy that is the basis for blood and urine pregnancy testing.

Hydrosalpinx: Obstruction of the fallopian tube at the fimbria, resulting in a fluid-filled and dilated tube.

Hyperprolactinemia: Excessive secretion of the hormone prolactin.

Hypoestrogenic: A state of low estrogen.

Hypo-osmotic swelling test: A sperm test that evaluates the integrity of the outer membrane of the sperm as a means to predict the sperm's fertilizing ability.

Hysterosalpingogram: An x-ray procedure during which a radio-opaque dye is injected into the uterine cavity to assess the fallopian tubes for patency as well as the contour of the uterine cavity itself.

Hysteroscopy: A procedure allowing visualization of the uterine cavity with a small fiber-optic telescope.

Hysterosonogram: A type of trans-vaginal sonogram performed after placement of a small catheter into the uterine cavity through which sterile water is introduced, allowing for visualization of the uterine cavity.

I

Implantation: The attachment of the early embryo to the endometrial lining of the uterus during the seventh to ninth days after ovulation.

Incompetent cervix: A muscular-fibrous weakening of the cervix, leading to painless cervical dilation and second-trimester or early third-trimester pregnancy loss.

Infertility: The inability of a couple to conceive after 12 months of unprotected intercourse.

Insulin resistance: Impaired response to insulin, which can lead eventually to diabetes.

Intracervical insemination: A fertility treatment in which sperm are placed within the cervix.

Intracytoplasmic sperm injection (ICSI): The injection of a single sperm into a single egg in an attempt to fertilize the egg in in vitro fertilization cases when fertilization might not otherwise occur.

Intrauterine adhesions: Fibrous bands of tissue found within the uterine cavity.

Intrauterine insemination (IUI): A fertility treatment in which the sperm are washed and then placed within the uterine cavity.

In vitro fertilization (IVF): A fertility treatment in which an egg is placed with a sperm cell in a laboratory culture dish, cultured for several days, and subsequently placed into the uterus.

K

Karyotype: The chromosomal complement of an individual, including the number of chromosomes and any chromosomal abnormalities.

L

Laparoscopy: An outpatient surgical procedure that uses a telescope and video monitor to visualize the internal organs.

Laparotomy: An inpatient surgical procedure that is performed through an open abdominal incision.

Luteal suppression: A stimulation protocol that involves suppression of the pituitary gland and ovary prior to initiating stimulation with fertility medications.

Luteinizing hormone (LH): A pituitary hormone that induces ovulation in a mature follicle.

M

Macroadenoma: A tumor of the pituitary gland measuring more than 1 cm.

Glossary

Menopause: The last menstrual period that a woman ever experiences.

Methyltetrahydrofolate reductase (MTHFR): An enzyme involved in folic acid metabolism.

Microadenoma: A tumor of the pituitary gland measuring less than 1 cm.

Monoamniotic twins: Monochorionic (identical) twins who share a single gestational sac. Carrying monoamniotic twins is considered to be a very high-risk pregnancy.

Monochorionic twins: Monozygotic twins who share a single placenta.

Monozygotic twins: Twins arising from a single fertilized egg (also called identical twins).

Morula: An early stage of embryonic development in which the embryo consists of a solid ball of cells; the morula is formed prior to the blastocyst.

Mosaicism: The presence of both genetically normal and abnormal cells within an embryo prior to implantation.

Mycoplasma: A type of bacteria that may contribute to infertility.

N

Natural Cycle IVF: IVF performed without the use of fertility medications and using the single follicle/egg that is produced in a regular reproductive cycle.

O

Oligospermia: An abnormally low concentration of sperm in a semen analysis.

Oral contraceptive pills: Daily medications, usually containing both synthetic estrogen and progesterone, that act as very effective contraceptives by suppressing follicle growth and ovulation.

Osteoporosis: Loss of calcium and bone mass, leading to an increased risk of fracture.

Ovarian hyperstimulation syndrome (OHSS): Ovarian enlargement, abdominal fluid retention, and dehydration following the use of fertility medication to induce the growth of multiple follicles.

Ovarian reserve: The fertility potential of a woman as determined by both the number of her ovarian follicles and the health of the eggs located within those follicles.

Ovary: A female reproductive organ that contains eggs within multiple follicles and produces reproductive hormones including estrogen and progesterone.

Ovulation: The release of an egg from an ovarian follicle.

Ovulation induction: The use of fertility medications to restore normal ovulation in a woman who does not have regular cycles.

P

Paracentesis: Placement of a needle through the abdominal wall so as to remove excess abdominal fluid.

Parvovirus B19: A virus that can cause an intrauterine infection leading to fetal anemia, fetal heart failure, and miscarriage.

Perimenopause: The years preceding the last menstrual cycle characterized by increasingly irregular cycles, hot flashes, and low estrogen levels.

Pituitary gland: An organ located at the base of the brain. It is often referred to as the "master gland" because it controls several of the other hormone-producing glands, including those responsible for metabolism and reproduction.

Polycystic ovarian syndrome (PCOS): A common gynecologic disorder resulting from insulin resistance and leading to irregular periods, acne, excessive facial hair, and infertility.

Postcoital test: A test of historical interest used to assess the presence and behavior of sperm found within the cervical mucus.

Preeclampsia: A vascular disease of pregnancy characterized by hypertension, edema, and a risk of seizure.

Preimplantation genetic diagnosis (PGD): Evaluation of the genetic status of an embryo prior to its implantation, usually through the removal of 1 to 2 cells at the 8-cell stage of development. The isolated cells can then be analyzed for specific chromosomal conditions and other genetic disorders.

Preimplantation genetic screening (PGS): An evaluation that is similar to preimplantation genetic diagnosis but is used to screen embryos in fertility patients for aneuploidy instead of a specific genetic disease.

Premature ovarian failure (POF): Irregular or absent menstrual cycles before the age of 40 years old, resulting from a marked loss of ovarian follicles as evidenced by a high blood level of follicle-stimulating hormone (FSH > 30 IU).

Progesterone: A steroid hormone produced by the ovary and then by the placenta during pregnancy. It is necessary for the successful implantation and development of an embryo.

Prolactin: A hormone produced by the anterior pituitary that stimulates breast milk production in a lactating woman. Inappropriate release of prolactin can cause irregular or absent menses.

Proteins C and S: Proteins involved in the blood clotting system.

Prothrombin II: A protein involved in the blood clotting system.

R

Reproductive endocrinologist: A physician who specializes in disorders of reproduction, including infertility.

Retrograde ejaculation: Backward movement of semen into the urinary bladder at the time of ejaculation.

S

Semen analysis: A laboratory test used to assess male fertility. It usually includes evaluation of the sperm volume, pH, concentration, motility and morphology in a sample.

Sperm Chromatin Structure Assay (SCSA®): A laboratory test used to determine the degree of DNA fragmentation within a sperm sample.

Sperm morphology: The shape and outward appearance of the sperm when viewed under a microscope.

Sperm motility: The movement of sperm when viewed under a microscope; it is usually expressed as a percentage of the sperm concentration.

Superovulation: The development of multiple ovarian follicles in response to fertility medication.

Systemic lupus erythematosus (lupus): A systemic autoimmune disease that causes inflammation, arthritis, rash, and other medical problems, including pregnancy loss.

T

Thrombophilia: A disorder of the blood clotting system resulting in a tendency to form blood clots. It may also lead to a higher risk of miscarriage.

Thyroid-stimulating hormone (TSH): A hormone produced by the pituitary gland that stimulates the production of thyroid hormone from the thyroid gland.

Transvaginal ultrasound: An imaging technique that uses sound waves produced by a wand-like probe placed within the vagina.

Trisomy: An abnormal genetic condition that arises when an individual possesses three copies of a particular chromosome instead of the normal two copies.

Tubal ligation: Surgical sterilization of a woman, performed by cutting or occluding the fallopian tubes.

Tubal reanastamosis: A surgical procedure to repair the fallopian tubes following a tubal sterilization procedure.

U

Ultrasonography: A noninvasive imaging technology that uses sound waves to create images of various structures in the body.

Ureaplasma: A type of bacteria that may contribute to infertility.

Uterus: The pear-shaped organ that contains a growing pregnancy; in lay terms, "the womb."

V

Varicocele: One or more dilated veins often located in the scrotal sac and thought to be a possible cause of male infertility.

Varicocelectomy: Ligation of dilated testicular or inguinal veins thought to be a source of male infertility.

Vasectomy: Surgical sterilization of a man by cutting the vas deferens.

Vitrification: An ultra-rapid method of freezing eggs and embryos that has dramatically improved the ability to cryopreserve unfertilized eggs and blastocyst stage embryos for future use.

W

Wyden law: Legislation passed by the U.S. Congress and sponsored by Congressman Ron Wyden that regulates the advertising and reporting of IVF success rates by fertility clinics.

X

X-linked recessive disease: A genetic disease associated with a mutation on the X chromosome. A male carrying such a mutation will have the disorder because he has only one X chromosome, but a female carrying a mutation on just one X chromosome has a normal gene on the other chromosome and so will not be affected by the disease.

Z

Zona pellucida: The outer cellular membrane that surrounds the egg and embryo up to the blastocyst stage of development.

Index

Index